NURSING HOME OPTIONS

Dr. Fisher's Guide . . .

NURSING HOME OPTIONS

Getting Quality Care for the Elderly

by

James Norman Fisher, M.D.

Collective Creations by Fisher
Publishers
Santa Barbara, California

Manufactured in the United States of America

Published by Collective Creations by Fisher

First printing 1991 by Kimberly Press, Inc.

Cover by J. B. Clark Graphics

LC: 91-073498

ISBN: 0-9629201-7-7: $9.25 Softcover

DEDICATION

This book is dedicated to a silver-haired Irish great-grandmother who grew to be ancient in years only. Sarah Carson Jackson taught me to respect the mind for what it is, the source of all inspiration and excitement, no matter its age. She lived 94 sparkling years and incited me to seek out those who had something to say of value. She entranced me with her stories, inviting me to careful listening.

It is also dedicated to the many past and present residents of Vista del Monte, the Retirement Home for California Teachers in Santa Barbara. I offer this work to honor them, being deeply indebted to the teaching profession for wonderful gifts of knowledge and opportunities to develop my own insights.

For over twenty-five years I have watched residents come and go, instructing me until the end. They never seemed to lose the need to communicate their feelings and wisdom as they walked paths before me, wishing to make my steps easier.

I can see them even now as I reflect on the memories of my days on "campus." They have been great friends and appreciative recipients of the many advices that they chose to seek from me. It has always been a great pleasure for me to serve them and enjoy their company.

ACKNOWLEDGEMENTS

I am deeply appreciative of those who have given much time and effort to reviewing this book. They include: Edward Steinfeldt, Consultant, Steinfeldt & Associates, Henry Holderman, M.D. and Kirk Gilbert, M.D., Family Physicians, Alan Gewant, Pharm. D., Nursing Home pharmacy provider, and Thelma Anderson and Harry Sootin, friends and patients.

Esther Slater has always been wonderful with her helpful suggestions since the early days at Goleta Valley Community Hospital.

Darwin Holian, M.D. was kind enough to spend many hours on his computer arranging this material into printer-ready documents.

And then there were three exceptional Directors of Nurses at Vista del Monte who through the years taught me much of what I know about Nursing Home care of the elderly—Elsie Bellefeuille, R.N., Nancy L. Fox, R.N., and Evelyn Bertanyi, R.N.

Much of the credit for any success of this book in improving care for the elderly belongs to these friends and colleagues.

DISCLAIMER

No discussion about Nursing Home care can consider every eventuality. The most common areas of concern are presented. A typical patient is everyone and no one at the same time. Each patient is a very individual case and requires very special consideration.

Moreover, each Nursing Home must comply with the standards of Federal, State, and County agencies, which by nature are separate and change frequently.

This material is not meant to answer specific legal questions. The legal documents referred to in the Appendices are examples only. Each State has its own set of recognized Advanced Directives. Please consult a knowledgeable attorney if you have questions.

It is not intended to weigh some of the moral issues involved. These areas are complex and very personal. Opinions expressed are solely those of the author.

This information is designed to guide you through what is for many a strange world of specialized care for the elderly. Having a personal relationship with your Family Doctor will help you make the right choices.

TABLE OF CONTENTS

ABOUT THE AUTHOR

James Norman Fisher was born in 1932 in Pittsburgh, Pennsylvania. He attended the University of Pittsburgh, graduating with a Bachelor of Science Degree in Bacteriology in 1954 and Doctor of Medicine Degree in 1958.

After interning in 1959 at Cottage Hospital in Santa Barbara, California, he served two years in the United States Air Force as a Flight Surgeon stationed in Korea. He married Betty Jean McBride in 1962 when he began practicing Family Medicine in Santa Barbara.

Since 1965 he has been the Medical Director of the Vista del Monte Retirement Home for California Teachers in Santa Barbara.

A founder of the Goleta Valley Community Hospital in 1966, he served as Board Chairman from 1973 until 1980.

Aside from his interest in Gerontology, he has been very active in the past in the American Academy of Family Physicians and the local chapter of the American Medical Association. He has two children and three grandchildren. His hobbies include genealogy, lapidary, piano, racquetball and hiking.

A fictional work, *And Into Death's Spiral*, the story of an AIDS Virus mutation plaguing the world in the late 1990's was published in 1990.

FOREWORD

Through the years I have spent many hours counseling patients and families about Nursing Homes. I have come to know what questions will usually be asked and what are the frequent concerns of caring relatives.

Especially facing the circumstances of "twilight time," the interval between a loved one's partial and complete dependence, it is crucial for families to gather information which can lead to a better understanding and evaluation of their options.

And because I've travelled with many elderly patients down the road to the end of their days, I feel this part of their life needs some open discussion. Family expectations are sometimes unrealistic. Misunderstandings are common. For those families who are suddenly confronted with a crisis, feelings may interfere with good judgment.

You will learn that as a patient or responsible family member there are many choices to make, more than you might imagine. **You are not at the mercy of others if you know your OPTIONS.**

What I will tell you is not written about or talked about very often in a particularly helpful way. Yet the advice I will give you has benefited many throughout the years. The concepts are simple. If there is a need to show love and affection to someone who needs support, my suggestions are easy to follow and apply.

For most patients, a lifetime of supporting others and being a responsible individual is poor preparation for being a dependent recipient. Roles are often reversed and are uncomfortable at first.

Yet, always the essential element is caring.

Nursing Home patients, or "**residents,**" as they are now called (I'll use both terms), are a very special challenge in communication. **And good communication is essential for good care.**

Those involved in caring should express their ideas so as to act in concert. That's not always possible, of course, but that is my goal as a physician and the goal of most families.

***NURSING HOME* OPTIONS** is meant to guide patients, family, responsible parties, and friends through the world of Nursing Home care from beginning to end. It will answer questions about **quality care** and what can be done to assure it.

The "**quality**" of any service, of course, is a personal judgment, each person being so unique in his preferences. Music, food, flowers, wine, etc.—we all have our particular likes and dislikes. We will look at the problems of measuring quality with the hope of finding something reasonably attainable for the resident about whom you are concerned.

Uncertain political clouds on the horizon will surely generate new **Options** in Nursing Home care. In fact, every aspect of the health care system, not just elder care, is currently under pressure to change. Present trends, costly and ineffective by many measures, cannot continue. Historically our Government has seemed helpless in managing our ever-increasing social demands. **There is a limit to social responsibility**. It may have already been exceeded, especially since taxation of working people is the usual solution. Practically, I can only address the present system and suggest ways and means to affect today's problems.

Certainly, Nursing Homes need to be held responsible to clients and their guardians who are charged by law to protect them. If there are Nursing Homes that provide poor and neglectful care, they are not alone in their blame. There must be a conspiracy of parties—families who don't or won't care, friends who will not speak up, professionals (doctors, nurses, aides, etc) who look the other way, administrators who view shabby methods as acceptable, inspectors at many levels (County, State, Federal) who file reports without expectation of corrective action, politicians who do not wish to highlight substandard services, public service groups, retirement groups, etc. who find it all too unimportant to warrant a vocal demonstration. Each and every one could make a great difference. **They certainly have other options.**

Those who exercise options about medical care must accept responsibility for those decisions and accept the consequences of their actions. That is part of the equation. Irresponsible action is worse than inaction.

Much of what I will say applies to medical care in a more general way and is helpful for that reason. These concepts are applicable in the acute hospital setting or in Geriatric Medicine. But my focus is on the Nursing Home. **I will highlight my suggestions and your choices as we go along.**

I like old folks. As a group, they are considerate and responsible, qualities that we see less frequently in younger generations. They are survivors, with many experiences from which we can learn. They have taught us much and can teach us more. They have earned and deserve assistance.

Though I have tried to view Nursing Home concerns in a general way, clearly these thoughts come through my eyes as a physician, one who has been responsible for seeing that my elderly friends are well taken care of. I cannot deny my prejudice to that end. Also, I admit to departing from conventional medical wisdom at times, a reflection of my personal experiences for over thirty years.

That residents of Nursing Homes will be treated appropriately and according to their wishes, particularly with dignity and respect, are my most important objectives.

Consider carefully the materials you will find here, for herein you may see your own future.

Respectfully,

James Norman Fisher, M.D.

INTRODUCTION

There is a roof, a very large roof, that reaches over every part of our country and covers more than 2.3 million greying heads each year, 1.5 million on any given day. It is shelter and home, providing food and family for a huge population of disabled.

Although wide media attention leads us often to think of the "homeless" who wander our streets, rarely do we consider the plight of "home-bound" Nursing Home residents. Without assistance they cannot manage the day-to-day business of living.

Having tried desperately to cling to ***independence***, they have unhappily succumbed to a life of ***dependence***, dependence on a family of nurses and assistants who comprise the Nursing Home setting. For financial support, they rely on their spouses, their family, their friends, their life savings and as a last resort, Federal and State Governments.

To be sure, for every patient the view is different but many of the essentials are the same.

estranged

Imagine yourself helpless—without the ability to walk, or talk or feed yourself or get to the bathroom. Yes! And maybe even blind and deaf and confused about where you are.

You are thrust into a **Nursing Home**, bedded down in a small room with a quiet stranger who seems always to be sleeping. Your cherished possessions are gone. You reach for a comb or a face cloth and nothing is there. Soon you are regimented to a life style that revolves around bodily function—eating, elimination, bathing, and sleeping. Your parents, spouse, peers—your companions of a lifetime—are gone. Rarely seeing the light of day, you are never alone or free to wander about. If accompanied, you may escape these walls only briefly.

This is how many perceive nursing home existence to be and there is much that applies.

Surely, only someone with many unfulfilled needs and few capabilities would voluntarily agree to live this way. Most submit because they cannot do otherwise or cannot comprehend such matters. Most are thankful to have somewhere to go—a place to carry on, a home where somebody cares. Repeating lifetime adaptations, they can learn to adjust to the schedule and find friendship in the faces around them. By doing so, they manage to hold on to a few more of life's precious moments.

When you've finished reading ***OPTIONS*** you will see beyond the surface, see what deeper needs are being satisfied here, recall the path that climaxes here, and consider alternatives. All along the way there are alternatives. Understanding those choices may make a great difference in how you deal personally with this aspect of life. Most families want and need a clearer appreciation of advanced aging.

For those who have no family or advocates, those who are separated from actuality, the problems are much greater. They are at the mercy of the system. The quality of their existence is likely to be a function of the most caring person nearby.

survivors

These are the same bright, red-cheeked, and cheerful faces that once ran through the schoolyard, grew to bear children of their own. They worked to support themselves and their community, eventually to find their spirit and strength slipping away. When we stumble in youth, we try to gain control of our balance. In the declining years we lose our equilibrium only to begin falling once again.

It is a path that more and more Americans are taking. It is a path that growing older provides. It is a path to the end of our days on earth—to the Nursing Home shelters that will become home to an increasing number of today's middle-aged Americans.

perspectives

Lest you think this is a gloomy and sad portrait, let me from the outset say that pleasure appears to be a matter of perspective.

A schoolchild might find Nursing Home circumstances quite restrictive and intolerable. In truth the process is often so subtle that those who live there may not find it so. Especially if those who are part of it, the Nursing Home staff, are able to bring cheer and warmth, friendship and love to bear.

This is a story about **good Nursing Home care**, about places where heads can come to rest to glean the last memories of a lifetime. Like every other phase of life there may be pain, but surely there is pleasure as well. It is that pleasure we wish to enhance. It is your part in that pleasure that I wish to encourage.

scope

In ***OPTIONS*** we will look briefly at the historical beginning of Nursing Homes and their evolution to include today's wide range of services. From the commonplace to elegant resort styles, we will examine their relationship to hospitals and the staff personnel that run them. Patient types, including typical medical problems, will be discussed to prepare you for the issues that will be presented later. The unique circumstances of **Alzheimer's Disease** are covered in a special chapter.

Dialogue about declining health, restraints, hospitalization, Cardio-Pulmonary Resuscitation, and the events that accompany dying are meant to condition you to be an effective agent when decisions need to be made.

Some of the issues of our day, the political, the religious, the social pressures that bear on the elderly, will be touched upon briefly.

In many ways we will approach the issues of **informed consent** and **self-determination**—the rights of patients and families to choose among the many options of care that are available. Both **PATIENT RIGHTS** and **THE PATIENT SELF-DETERMINATION ACT** are legislative efforts to regulate consent for medical treatments.

Lastly, one chapter on **Advanced Directives** will afford some ideas about protecting "**BODYRIGHTS**," the rights each of us has to protect the body when the brain can no longer maintain control.

an open mind

Begin reading with an open mind and an open spirit. Reach inside, not only to find your own thoughts about the precious few moments we call life, but look as well to find the meaning that others find. **Perspectives change for all of us as we grow.**

I've found that there is no polite way to advise people about aging or its problems. Our own aging seems always to cloud the way we view the future. Certainly, these are very sensitive areas. For after all there is no proper way to grow old, no truly graceful process. We tumble often as we try. Foresight is helpful but not consistently effective in preventing catastrophe. Best intentions are forever being thwarted by reality. **Being willing to accept events and circumstances that are not easily controlled, is one way to cope.**

Please use the full range of ***OPTIONS*** for patients and families and close friends. Choose ones that can enrich the lives of those who need your support.

Chapter 1

WHY THIS PLACE?

the road that leads us

In the beginning the "Whys" of Nursing Home care are all tough questions. Why now? Why me? Why are you doing this to me? Why can't I stay for a while longer where I am?

A strong desire for self-control provokes the same questions at every juncture of life. Beginning in childhood, independent characters mouth them with increasing stubbornness, right to the end.

Coming to advanced maturity is a large generation of Twentieth Century Americans. They have benefited by a host of scientific break-throughs, resulting in unprecedented numbers becoming grandparents and great-grandparents. They are on the edge of a new frontier—**the frontier of aging in the modern world.**

Never before have so many been given the gift of time—more time to circle the sun and enjoy the rewards of a lifetime of productive labor. Not that humans today are capable of living longer than our ancestors, but in our modern era more actually survive the hazards, pushing life expectancy higher and higher.

Forty million people will have become eligible for Medicare benefits before 1992, most having passed their 65th birthday.

Upon graduation from work they look forward to travel, recreation, a retirement income and the pleasures of their grandchildren. Quite incidentally, they encounter the real prospect of "ripe old age."

Looking at the group over 65, we must be impressed with their energy and youthfulness. Their accomplishments and experiences are vast and remarkable. Like teenagers, they concentrate on today and what's happening now. Most find the thought of their life ever coming to an end a premature notion, the mind noting little of the deterioration that the rest of the body feels much earlier.

winding down

Although they have begun to limit possessions, move to a smaller retirement setting, wind down busy schedules, and enjoy more recreation, most never consider the strong likelihood of spending time in a Nursing Home. That's not only unrealistic, but also a bit of foolish

Table 1 LIVING ARRANGEMENTS

Private Family Living
- family home
- apartment
- mobile home
- farm
- home equity conversions
- adapted quarters

Community Living
- shared housing
- congregational living
- condos

Planned Community Living
- retirement centers
- ECHO (granny flats)
  (elderly cottage housing opportunity)
- continuing care retirement community

Health Care Centers
- custodial care
- board and care
- personal care units
- intermediate care
- assisted living
- acute hospitals
- rehabilitation centers
- skilled nursing (SNF)

optimism. For 30% will live there—on average more than two years. Most of these will die there.

The path that will lead there is an elusive and deceptive one. If they are graced with hereditary longevity, it is almost inevitable. They will experience advanced old age and a Nursing Home. Dreamers may avoid the thought for a time but not the reality.

By the end of this century in the U.S.A. there will be almost 5 million people over the age of eighty-five, the most vulnerable and dependent years. Today we house 20% of this group in Nursing Homes.

In a society of free individuals, confinement is an unthinkable notion. The achievement of freedom is one of the paramount goals of a lifetime, once attained, not easily given up. Yet, as a matter of fact, those things we strive to do, the accomplishments of our youthful days, are the things that one-by-one we surrender to old age.

Moreover, families are very reluctant to place their parents in Nursing Homes because of a sense of abandonment. Though they cannot cope with the many frailties of aging, there is guilt about their inadequacy, only one of many psychological barriers to a Nursing Home admission.

when help is needed

The transition from helping to being helped has usually a gentle beginning. Rather than providing for our own needs, we look to others. One thing after another is done by someone else. Little by little, we give up self-control, self-sufficiency.

Once the children are grown, independent family living is easily traded for a less tedious, less expensive life style. Most older couples enjoy walking away from responsibility toward simpler patterns.

Table 1 shows the common pathways for those who survive, each level more dependent than the one before. Circumstances of health and finances, as well as social situations, sweep people along as they age. New settings are added to the list everyday, giving today's retired generations many more choices.

Springing out of the social accomplishments of our time, is a network of support services to pick up when help is needed. **Table 2** lists the services that most communities can provide.

TABLE 2 SERVICES AVAILABLE IN THE COMMUNITY

TABLE 2 SERVICES AVAILABLE IN THE COMMUNITY
County Information and Referral Services
Community Health Clinics
Emergency Assistance Crisis Intervention
Advocacy/Legal Services
Visiting Nurses
Hospice
Intravenous Home Therapy
Aids and Assistive Devices
Community Action Groups
Nutrition Sites
Home Health care
Volunteer Visitors
Live-in Companion
Family Respite Service
Foster Grandparents
Meals on Wheels
Night Sitters
Shopping Aides
Care giver Support Groups
Readers for Partially Sighted
Chauffeured Transportation
Self-help Volunteer Programs
Grocery Deliveries
Telephone Contact
Senior Centers
Foster Home
Share-a-Home
Day Care
Laundry Services
High School Programs
In-home Equipment
Lay Health Organizations

The usual health care providers within the community include the physician, physician's assistant, nurse practitioner, social worker, home health aide, occupational therapist, and physical therapist.

Those who live alone can often continue in that setting with the help of these outside services. However, close monitoring is essential to avoid a crisis in these situations. Those who provide assistance are often first to discover other needs.

There are Retirement Centers arising all across the country. They provide living arrangements designed expressly for those who are growing older. At the same time, they coordinate the services listed and oversee others. The costs are usually reasonable.

in-home nursing

Most communities have two outstanding resources that have come of age in recent years to provide excellent home nursing care—The Visiting Nurses Association (VNA) and Hospice. Both are constantly expanding their services.

The VNA offers home care for many kinds of situations which might otherwise require the Hospital or Nursing Home. They can follow up on in-patient treatments to enable patients to return home sooner. Medical doctors have found them to be of invaluable assistance.

Hospice is organized to treat terminal cancer patients and other terminally ill patients such as those with AIDS, giving them the option to spend their last days at home. They have many support group services as well. Patients and families are very appreciative.

health care centers

Whatever the progression of needs, each is clearly a step backward for the patient who loses more and more private choices. Some resist every step of the way. Some willingly accept. Last on everyone's list are health care centers. Of those, the Skilled Nursing Home level provides the most long-term assistance.

It's not always the end of the line. Fortunately, many are rehabilitated there. After an initial Hospital stay, followed by Nursing Home therapy, they are returned home or to another level of care.

Hospitals, service organizations and private groups are constantly looking to create less expensive ways to preserve independence. Government has for some time been funding such efforts.

concepts of medical dependence

From a medical perspective there are only two kinds of dependence, either **physical or mental**. We become dependent on someone's physical ability to do something for us, or their mental capability to help us solve a problem. Of course, these are rarely isolated problems, but thinking about dependence as two separate entities helps us sort out solutions.

Table 3 shows the regression from both physical and mental independence to total dependence. Just before a patient becomes totally dependent, there is what I call "twilight time," when crises tend to happen, alerting us to the need for special attention.

Some kinds of disability are carefully plotted out on a scale of numbers and letters. This is mostly for the sake of compensation payments, such as Worker's Compensation. The American Heart Association has such a scale for rating heart disease. The scientific appraisal of disability is a tool which has become more sophisticated, more carefully defining the ranges of limitations.

Physical weakness comes in many varieties and for many different medical reasons. **Mental decline** is also varied and often is associated with confusion. They are not always parallel, nor are their patterns

TABLE 3 CONCEPTS OF MEDICAL DEPENDENCE

PHYSICAL	MENTAL	LEVEL OF FUNCTION
		INDEPENDENT
strong	bright	healthy productive
		PARTIAL DEPENDENCE
weak	slow	help needed
* * * TWILIGHT TIME * * *		
		TOTAL DEPENDENCE
very weak	confused	helpless

distinctive. Most Nursing Home patients are of mixed disability, **but they are all dependent.**

twilight time

Somewhere between partial independence and complete dependence is a "twilight time." It is the vulnerable time, sometimes brief, sometimes long, a hanging-on time, when the surrounding support systems are sorely tested. Help may be available and useful. At other times, patients make do or work their way around the problem so as to maintain control without visible assistance.

More and more efforts are being directed at assisting the "twilighters." But as family life becomes more disrupted, as mobility has increased for offspring, as fewer couples live together, as spouses and family pass on, more of the elderly live alone. Close friends are fewer. Families have a much harder time looking after one another. Children find it difficult to direct their parents.

For families it becomes a time of "one-way bargaining." Determined matriarchs tell everyone how it will be, no matter that they are becoming a severe burden to so many. Clear reasoning is impossible. Good judgment is lacking. Unreasonable expectations can lead to family conflict and strain, hence to a crisis. Some communities have a Geriatric Crisis Team available to assist where there is a serious risk to health.

Waiting for something to happen can be exasperating but is often the only approach some families can use.

A serious acute illness can temporarily disable even the youngest and strongest. But in "twilight time," minor illness can totally disable. The thin edge makes it easy to trip, if no one is there to catch them.

There are many levels of assistance in Health Care Centers to be considered before the Skilled Nursing Home level. The question is always, "which will suffice for now and when is the Skilled Nursing Facility absolutely necessary?"

a falling out, a falling down

Falling out of step where others can notice, will lay open the vulnerability that may have been hidden, the social interaction that had been avoided. Other problems will emerge.

Unfortunately, the crisis that develops often results in hospitalization. There the Social Service department sorts out the available information and attempts to find a solution. Nursing Home placement is often part of the chain of settings that establishes a new life style.

Chapter 11 will discuss the most common ailments seen in a Nursing Home. **They are in fact the reasons why most patients are there in the first place.** They include incontinence, confusion, and falling.

In planned communities where various levels of care are available, many requirements for independent living are mandated by law (Fire and Safety Codes). Several kinds of assessments are used by management to determine when a patient needs more help or needs to move to a higher level of care. These are based on in-depth evaluations of each of the **Activities of Daily Living (ADL)** and are usually scored. The resulting determination is very helpful for all concerned, being the scientific way of assessing disability and functional needs.

a life line

Dependent individuals would not survive long without life support. Life is sustained only by the grace of others.

Impossible in the animal world, this is possible in our world for two reasons: human emotional attachment and the application of accumulated resources. This group of patients then are living with their own financial resources or by the grace of their benefactors. In primitive societies they would succumb to tribal customs.

In our society when dependent individuals become disconnected, isolated, and adrift, they are sustained in a specially created, artificial world of support systems. It is no wonder then that the Nursing Home setting is so foreign to most visitors. As common as Nursing Homes are, they are in a sense quite unnatural, a phenomenon of the new frontier of aging.

the giant step

Stepping inside a Nursing Home is the giant step that everyone avoids. But one way or another, one time or another, eventually it happens.

A major crisis is the direct way, the most common way, in effect the easy way to enter a Nursing Home. Once admitted, it is not easy to be released without proving competence. Too many eyes can focus on the consequences of a misstep, the risks of independent living.

Voluntary admissions are the hardest, most wrenching admissions. These are the patients whose problems culminate in a conscious decision. Carried, in a wheelchair, or walking in, patients express a host of feelings, depending on what they expect. Earlier preparation will be helpful if the mind can comprehend and remember.

Family and friends are as much affected as the patient because they think they know more about what might happen. They dread the thoughts of a Nursing Home existence. Like the first day of school, apprehension is the great bugaboo.

Most patients actually acclimatize incredibly soon, unless something harsh happens to frighten them. In a week's time, and often sooner, many feel and act like they have been there for years. Time takes on a new dimension.

SUMMARY:

Today, Americans are living longer and expect medical technology to continue to preserve their modern life style. Sooner or later, many begin to lose independence, and although postponed by a variety of support services, at last find Nursing Homes their final residence. There they live in an unnatural setting, continuing beyond their mental and physical ability to cope. They accept the Nursing Home process and become ***pioneers in the Aging Frontier****.*

OPTIONS:

- It is easier to find assistance when there is no urgency. Plan ahead to avoid a crisis.
- Accept the notion that one day you or a loved one will need more help. Choose a setting where help is available.
- Accept help when it is appropriate and beneficial to health and well being. Rely on the family, the doctor, and good friends. Be willing to alter lifestyles in order to maximize rewards and pleasures.
- Look for new interests in new surroundings. Anticipating a disastrous experience will not be helpful.

Chapter 2

HOME

a rocking chair by the fireplace

> It may not be much, just the essentials. A bed and a bath, some common areas, a dining room, a recreation room, a garden, and maybe a chapel—but it's home. And life goes on

Most of us picture old age as we would like it to be. Maybe a porch and a rocking chair, or a fireplace, certainly cozy and warm. The movies manage it very well, rarely touching on the details of "fading away," as some think of it.

But "fading away" is indeed a very complicated process, one that more and more often occurs away from home, in Hospitals or Nursing Homes, out of view of close family. But what kind of places are these facilities? Where did they come from? What have they become?

in the old days

Today our elderly are abundant, a by-product of industrial and scientific advancement. But not long ago there were very few "old-timers." The rugged individuals who did survive were revered and respected.

In agrarian societies like early America, the aged were segregated only if they were poor or destitute. They were gathered into "poor houses" or "alms houses" where public funds made a gesture of humanitarian assistance. Being needy was not a respectable condition. The crippled and insane were included with them.

For those who could afford care and whose family assisted, there were established "homes," usually small and private, where a widow or poor family took on the job of caretaker.

Doctors were unnecessary. Their talents were not particularly beneficial to those within, whose problems were not really "medical" in nature. Patients received supportive non-medical care.

Other cultures managed aging in their own way. On the opposite side of the globe the Chinese adopted what came to be known as "Death Houses." They were shelters for the sick and needy where food was provided daily for those who could reach and eat, a clear impossibility for most. Hence the name.

The Eskimos once removed the elderly to a remote area of the frozen wilderness where hypothermia would peacefully end their days.

Tribal cultures as a rule sought out "natural" ways for the elements to overtake the frail and the unproductive.

changing attitudes

Common to most religions, a deep desire to protect the needy changed the way disability was viewed. With the advances of modern medicine and economic prosperity, not only could life-threatening illness be cured but function could be restored as well. Patients, even the elderly, could return to former activities.

Then, in America during the 1930's came the Great Society concept which ushered in new social systems. Social Security was born. It was a pension fund managed by the Government, which never considered nor intended that retirement proceeds might ever be used for the feeble aged. But like most of the benefits which issued from Washington's social consciousness, their scope became far greater and considerably more costly than planners had ever imagined.

Rejuvenation has become common place. With sophistication of medical treatments and by pooling resources (insurance), patients expected full treatment and every effort to return them to recovery. As the per-day cost of hospital care soared, other facilities were developed for less intense convalescent care. Nursing Homes found a new impetus after WWII.

Gradually then, the small private "nursing home" became a "convalescent home," became an "extended care facility," became a "skilled nursing facility." Licensing has stiffened the requirements for every kind of elder care.

In today's changing society we continually find newer concepts of treatment coming into being. So too, attitudes about recovery have changed, influencing the length of treatments and their outcome. Technology has been critical in the evolution of today's Nursing Home. Many have become specialized rehabilitation centers where long and complex treatments are given.

a new industry

In the 1990's, a **Skilled Nursing Facility (SNF)** is the ultimate in long-term nursing care institutions. It provides highly-specialized nursing care of all kinds to very dependent patients. The Government defines the kinds of nursing skills which constitute Medicare and Medicaid approved benefits.

Intermediate Care Facility (INF) is a term once used to indicate a lesser level of nursing care but it is seldom used any longer. **Custodial**

Care does not involve skilled nursing care and such care is usually regulated by local governments.

Most of today's Nursing Homes have been built since 1967, soon after Medicare came into being.

Entrepreneurs moved in to fill a need. Government funding supported the boom. Both non-profit and for-profit institutions can be found.

With Medicare, the "medical nature" of the Skilled Nursing Home was clearly and securely established. Eligibility was predicated on a medical diagnosis, determined by a physician. Treatment reflected his "orders."

types of patients

After twenty-five years of adjustment and reform, Skilled Nursing Homes presently serve **three principle functions**:

—a residence for the feeble elderly;

—a recovery and therapy setting for acutely ill patients after treatment in hospitals en route to returning home or to another setting;

—a death bed for the terminally ill who have become unmanageable at home.

Not always distinct, each category has its particular management problems.

The first group, **the feeble elderly**, are in sheer numbers the most prominent sector. These are the long-term custodial cases. For the most part, they have exhausted Medicare benefits, used up private resources and now are receiving Medicaid (State and Federal financing). They have chronic medical conditions with little or no hope of moving out.

The second group, **the acutely ill**, is much like the first except that they have acute problems from which they are recovering. **Medicare** is usually footing the bill and scrutinizing the care. The goal is to return them to their homes or previous settings. But because each setback takes away some further degree of independence, many will not return. This level of Nursing Home care is higher, requiring more treatments, i.e. Physical Therapy, Speech Therapy, Occupational Therapy, etc. When progress is limited or they relapse, these patients become part of the first group.

The last group, **the terminally ill**, is a difficult treatment group. Often they are supported in various ways, sometimes prolonging their lives with efforts at nutritional balance, fluids, antibiotics, etc. The demand for bedside nursing care can be very great.

There is one other general group of Nursing Home residents. This is **the younger set**. They have Muscular Dystrophy, Multiple Sclerosis, severe injuries, etc. AIDS has added still another new population of the young. Disabled early in life, they live under the same roof with the elderly and in many instances go through the same kinds of experiences.

These four categories, although quite different in requirements for care, are mixed together in most Nursing Homes.

Not included are primary psychiatric cases who defer to psychiatric facilities. **Mental disorders within Nursing Homes are organic, i.e. diseases resulting from actual brain damage**.

specialty care

Of course, there are specialty Nursing Homes that have one particular service to perform, i.e. stroke rehabilitation, spinal cord rehabilitation, cardiac rehabilitation, Alzheimer's Disease, etc.

Like hospitals, many Skilled Nursing Facilities are sponsored by churches, service clubs, charitable organizations, veterans' groups, auto workers and other labor groups. Qualifying for one or another of these can be a tremendous benefit to a patient, not only financially but because of the camaraderie that a common background will provide. Insurance packages sometime include such care.

Considering all the types of Nursing Homes, you can see that the roof I spoke of is indeed wide and varied, in size, location, access, and character.

accoutrements

While some Nursing Homes are posh, some are pitiful. The range is very wide although the basic services to be provided are meant to be similar, being reimbursed in similar ways and regulated by the same Government agencies.

In a free society some people live in squalor as a way of life. Newspapers tell of the horrors of filthy Nursing Homes. The worst scenarios make the headlines, revealing smelly, crowded, understaffed conditions and unkempt patients with bed sores, and sometimes patients subjected to bad food and abuse. Even the words conjure the worst of Hell's nightmares—snakepits of survival. This is one extreme.

State-of-the-art "homes" include giant screen television, recreation halls, private telephones, gardens, courtyards, bus transportation, and consortium accommodations.

Most good Nursing Homes rely on word-of-mouth referrals and a good image within the community. And in fact, personal references may be your best source of information about a facility. Ask around your community.

making a choice

In **the triangle of Nursing Home care,** there are three pillars: the Home itself, the family, and the doctor. The Nursing Home is crucial in the quality of care. The facility must be functional, the staff qualified and devoted. The role of the family and doctor will be described later.

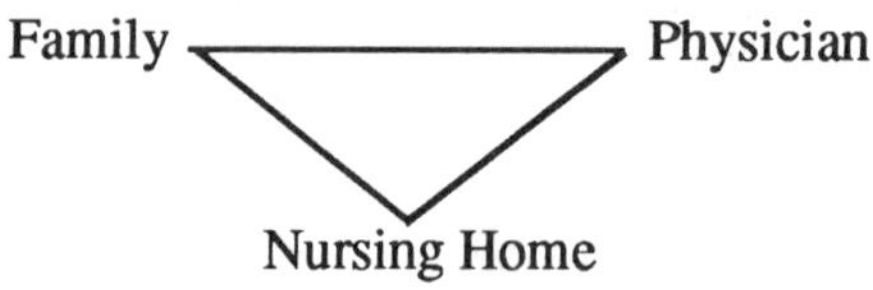

There are pages and pages of standards that inspectors review when they critique a Nursing Home, meant to identify serious or potentially-serious risks to patients. Their reports are sometimes filled with petty "deficiencies" which can be very slight deviations from complex legislative requirements. These reports are required to be posted in all facilities and are available for public review.

Your pick of a Nursing Home should be made on the tangible and visible evidences of "good care" and other compelling considerations. No matter how many charts you construct to rate Nursing Homes, it comes down to rather simple assessments and gut feelings. These characteristics of a Nursing Home stand out above the others in importance:

- **cleanliness and condition of patients**
- **location, convenience to family**
- **the Director of Nurses**
- **the staff—kindness and length of service**
- **food**
- **services available (depends on the individual case)**
- **cost**
- **personal reasons**

—No matter what part of the country, no matter how remote from town, no matter how antiquated the roof, **the place must be clean.** This is the most important test of Nursing Home care. Not just the floors and tables and chairs, but the patients. Clothes get worn and tousled, but residents should look clean and be free of odor. An abundance of linen is one good indication of cleanliness. Health care workers should certainly have a neat appearance.

—The location is very important to family members who will be visiting frequently. Convenient access is very helpful to close supervision.

—I will discuss the importance of the Director of Nurses, the DON, in coming chapters. As the critical person in the Nursing Home, he/she must satisfy your expectations as a competent, interested, and caring person.

—A good staff remains in place and employees are faithful. Where faces change from month to month, the management approach must be questioned.

—The food that is served in institutions finds it hard to compete with home cooking. But it should be nutritionally adequate, appealing and well presented.

—There may be other personal reasons that are important to you that deserve careful evaluation such as services available and cost. But remember, **there is no perfect place, no perfect solution, just as there is no perfect patient**.

Unfortunately most Nursing Homes admissions are not by choice. An acute medical emergency, often an injury, sets families scrambling for a Nursing Home bed. Social Service personnel come into action, providing lists of currently available places. Often there is little time to choose carefully.

SUMMARY:

Social programs have provided new standards of living for the feeble elderly in this country. Patients have more options if they choose a Nursing Home of their liking with a philosophy similar to their own and where the quality of care is apparent.

OPTIONS:

- Choose Nursing Home care only when all other possibilities are exhausted.
- Ask yourself what you expect to accomplish with Nursing Home care, the types of services you will need.
- If specialized institutional care is available, explore those possibilities.
- Use common sense as you make judgments about Nursing Homes. The quality of care is usually very obvious. Choose the Nursing Home that will function best for you.

Chapter 3

THE CAST

the staff in action

> You should know the cast of players if you are to understand the play. In Nursing Home life each character has a part. The performance is smooth if everyone knows his role and what's expected of the others.

Good management sends out strong signals about primary purpose and other important objectives.

To provide necessary nursing care to residents is the essential reason for the existence of all Nursing Homes. Everyone in the institution must know that.

hospital model

As Nursing Homes expanded to provide post hospital care, they became more and more like them. What before was little more than a bed and breakfast became an extension of the hospital. It is not surprising then that the organization of a Nursing Home is fashioned after the hospital industry which it closely mirrors.

From the ward setting, the therapy rooms, the kitchen, to the business office, they look very much alike. On the patient service side, 2-3 bed rooms are organized into 20-30 bed wards, usually a wing, with central nursing stations. Nearby will be a dining room, some recreation areas, gardens, and patios. Treatment areas are usually at hand. The service areas, a kitchen, a house cleaning department and a maintenance department are secreted somewhere on the premises. Large institutions may have such capabilities at a distance. Administrative services are much less noticeable because there is usually little turnover of patients and much less bookkeeping than in a hospital. This is changing somewhat, however, as hospitals move patients out earlier.

Patients congregate for meals. One room commonly serves as a dining room and a recreation room.

Physicians' offices in Nursing Homes are unusual but rehabilitation facilities, Occupational Therapy and Physical Therapy, are common, depending on the demand for such programs.

If the Nursing Home is part of a larger retirement complex, then it may be blessed with many "campus features," i.e. libraries, beauty shops, hobby or craft areas, pool halls, swimming pools, visitors' facilities and a private view of paths and gardens. More importantly, close friends may be near for support.

the performers

Patient care is provided principally by nurses, aides and orderlies who have been trained in hospitals.

Although 90% of patient contact is actually provided by aides and orderlies, the ward nurse is the overseer. She and her staff are the working unit.

The Director of Nurses, or DON, is the operations officer. She (most are women) is responsible for everything that happens, supervising all the nurses, each and every shift. The Director of Staff Development helps train the staff. Together they perform many functions related to quality control.

At some distance is the Owner /Board of Directors who manages the system via the Administrator, who oversees not only all of the Medical services but all departments, including Administration, Housekeeping, Dietary, and Maintenance. The Medical Director serves a supportive role for the Administrator and the DON. I will discuss these three important positions in separate chapters to follow.

Unlike hospitals, doctors are seldom in evidence as their visits are ordinarily once each month. Occasionally, the Medical Director will be seen when he attends his own patients or visits with the staff.

cross connections

Organizational charts are an easy way to visualize the operation of the system. Please refer to the Organizational Chart in **Appendix A** to see how each department relates to the other.

Vital to a smooth performance is the way information moves between departments and the teamwork of the leaders. Some institutions operate at the bottom without much direction from above. Others follow the orders from on high and pay little attention to the problems of the lower echelon. **Freely flowing information and problem solving in both directions are essential for smooth institutional functioning and ultimately good patient care**.

duties

The duties of the principal characters are listed in the job descriptions in **Appendix B**. They are spelled out so you may become familiar with the responsibilities each has in the chain of care giving.

licensing

Nursing Homes are licensed by a number of agencies who monitor their activities. These include Federal, State, and Local Government.

Transfer Agreements between Hospitals and Nursing Homes are required as patients are moved between them, part of certification and reimbursement eligibility.

As requirements have broadened, more and more categories of personnel are licensed as well. Additional training for all employees has been mandated by law in several areas of job performance.

"together"— the team approach

Each facility and staff attempt to present an image of togetherness. They see themselves as part of a family whose function it is to provide very complete and personal services to the paying resident.

Color-coordinated uniforms and name badges are meant to keep residents from being confused. They identify roles for residents and visitors.

Teams are organized to perform functions, allowing one member to support another when special problems arise. That takes the pressure off of individuals and improves the atmosphere for workers. Good teams are proud of their collective effort.

SUMMARY:

Each Nursing Home has its staff of highly trained and licensed personnel. Organizationally they are similar to Hospitals but their individual approach to problems can be very different. To effectively use the many services available, a patient advocate needs to know the hierarchy of personnel and their roles, and should interact, one-on-one, with as many levels as possible.

OPTIONS:

- Become familiar with members of the staff and their roles. Take time to meet them individually.
- First names will bring you closer to the care givers, making you part of their family.
- Take the position of asking questions rather than giving advice or direction. The responder is more likely to become a teaching advocate, a position of respect, than to feel like the object of criticism.
- Brief notes to those involved in care will show your interest and make you someone to be reckoned with and satisfied.

Chapter 4

THE DON

the director of nurses

> She is the essential force behind all nursing activity. Most Nursing Homes reflect her personality and strength. Not unlike the structure of any family group, one person assumes responsibility for the well being of all dependents as a personal challenge. Although men perform as DON's, the essence of their functioning is maternal and caring and reassuring.

There is a special breed of nurses that supervise Nursing Homes. Up from the ranks, or occasionally moving from acute-care Hospitals or clinics, comes the Director of Nurses, better known as the DON. She is the warmest and most caring of professionals.

the character

In this particular setting, only certain spirited personalities can remain strong over a long period of time. The reasons are simple. The DON must establish long-term relationships with patients who seldom return to robust good health. She must be cheerful and outgoing and attentive to those who often are not able to reciprocate, sometimes not even able to respond. She must be supportive and strong in an industry where the staff in all departments is changing constantly and many new workers need to be trained and observed again and again. To the residents of Nursing Homes she is a true "Angel of Mercy."

the job

First and foremost, she "nurses the nurses." There is much need for hand holding here for reasons you will discover. There must be a shoulder to come to, a source of information and support. Without that, the turnover of nurses becomes excessive.

She must know every job thoroughly. It is the only way she can provide answers to numerous questions that arise daily. Occasionally, she will fill in for one who is absent.

Being the principal coordinator, knowing the families of patients is an fundamental part of her role. She wants to meet responsible family members and to understand their feelings. When crises arise, her presence is reassuring to everyone involved.

As a rule, she is the one person most knowledgeable about all aspects of a case. Factors outside the institution, social situations, etc., which interrelate with what happens inside the facility will be known to her. She is the most consistently-available character in a Nursing Home.

Of course she is responsible to the Administrator, but all nursing-related activities seem to spring from her role. She is consulted by the attending physician, the support services, the many therapists, families, etc. All come to her desk for answers. She delegates authority and some responsibilities but must be aware of them all.

She must be a manager as well as a nurse. Rules and regulations fill her life. Every report related to the Nursing Home crosses her desk. Every incident involving a resident or employee is submitted to her for comments and\or action.

Because Federal and State regulations are ever changing, the DON must be aware of the latest standards of care as well as remain current as a Registered Nurse. She attends innumerable meetings both in and out of the Nursing Home in order to keep up.

professionalism

You will see the pride and poise of a professional Registered Nurse in the DON. Indeed, she has reached a high degree of competence to achieve her status. Long hours of solving problems have led her to this level of responsibility. Very few can manage the scope of her activities and knowledge.

She recognizes the importance of all disciplines and will usually emphasize the team approach. Her reliance on other members of the staff and their recognition of her role creates harmony that translates into good patient care.

"touching"

Any DON who cannot be seen touching patients is probably not a good communicator and may well be having difficulty with her job. She must seek out that side of her job to assure herself that her efforts are effective. Family concerns must be attended as well. She should show a genuine interest in you as a family member.

problems of the DON

To begin with, her salary is lower than most comparable positions in hospitals or private settings. Were it not for a special interest in the elderly and the needs of these residents, she could be content to serve her profession in a 40-hour-week salaried position.

All the problems of the Nursing Home are problems of the DON.

Frustrations are many. There is pressure to meet budgets. Limited by one of the lowest wage scales in any industry, she frequently has to call for "registry help," or "on call" temporary personnel from local job agencies. Not only do costs escalate rapidly but then every shift has changing faces for patients to find each day, disrupting the continuity of care.

The high pressure, quick decisions, fast-action problems of the acute-care hospital nurse are replaced by the slower pace and more routine activities. But the psychological demands of work are more telling than they seem. Severe and depressing events occur often. Patient progress is slow or more often declining. The importance of a "thank you," a smile, a pat on the back, cannot be underestimated. These gestures bring renewed effort.

other nurses on staff

I do not wish to minimize the roles of other staff nurses, RN's, LVN's, and CNA's, who share many of the same problems and must be equally dedicated to patients.

Most of these nurses also come from the acute-care setting or hospital and therefore are older and more experienced. They feel many of the same stresses that I have described for the DON.

Know the nurses and staff that attend your family member. Treat them humanely and they will respond in kind. If you can, help them with simple chores, getting water or walking patients, and you can become part of the team.

hands-on care

Aides and orderlies are responsible for the actual hands-on care within the Nursing Home. They are critical in the administration of **quality care**. This is something a good DON never forgets and takes personal pride in. She prizes staff members who give that extra personal touch.

Those who work as attendants are **usually working two jobs,** sometimes three. Under such stress, workers frequently do not "show up" for duty. Absenteeism is high. Often coming from minority groups within the community, they may speak foreign languages among themselves which can be disorienting for elderly residents who hear them.

territories

Remember that life is a game of territories. Those who are insecure tend to guard their prerogatives carefully, object to change, and demand respect from those who enter their domain. Understand territories and you can be very helpful.

Your respect for those who are trying hard to be efficient will permit you to pass through "their space" without a scene.

Begin to interfere with schedules and routines and their feeling toward you might be converted to misgivings about the patient. It behooves you to be cooperative.

Medical personnel want to be liked and respected. They respond with graciousness. On the other hand, arrogance on the part of an unappreciative family is a sure road to conflict.

If you think of those who treat residents as an extension of your family, forgetting prejudice and pettiness, and think of the overall effort—you will surely get better care for grandma or grandpa.

SUMMARY:

The most critical personality in a Nursing Home is the Director of Nurses. She is the hub of activity. Understand her problems and you will better be able to support her, and will be more likely to receive ***quality care*** *for your loved one.*

OPTIONS:

- Befriend the DON, the most important person in the Nursing Home other than your loved one.
- On a day-to-day basis the charge nurse can answer most all of your questions. Seek her out when you have problems.
- Actually everyone you can befriend will touch your resident where it counts the most, on a one-to-one basis, each and every day.
- Appreciate the work of aides and orderlies. The rest of the nursing staff know how important they really are.

Chapter 5

THE HEALTH CARE ADMINISTRATOR

the chief executive officer

> Representing the Owner or the Board of Directors, he is the general manager of all Nursing Home business, often behind the scenes.

The person responsible for **everything** that goes on in a Nursing Home is the Health Care Administrator. All the important positions within a Nursing Home have been filled by him.

He is the ultimate authority about Nursing Home care. Trained with on-the-job experience and licensed by the State, he is well qualified to have such responsibility.

ownership

Ownership may be private or corporate where management is comprised of a Board of Directors. Chosen by the owner/board to carry out policies, the Administrator represents them both to residents and the public.

the character

Wide and varied backgrounds are found among Nursing Home Administrators. Managing people is the prime prerequisite. Turning a profit is essential. Medical knowledge and social skills are part of the package.

Most use the team concept, meeting regularly with department heads and consultants. They usually chair in-house committee meetings such as the Utilization Review Committee, Fire Safety Committee, and Quality Assurance Committee. Minutes are kept to document the proceedings.

The Quality Assurance Committee is the instrument by which Nursing Homes insure **quality care**. There are many mechanisms by which services can be assessed. This committee is mandated to evaluate patient care on a regular basis, specifically addressing the issues of patient rights and the quality of life.

Public relations are an important part of the Administrator's function. He wants to run a good facility and meet all the requirements of regulators. He also wants to know what residents and their families think about his team.

the job

Much of the Administrator's time is devoted to seeing that his institution complies with legal mandates.

In California there is **Title 22** which has been the guiding light of Nursing Home care for almost 10 years now, upon which Federal directives have been modeled.

Then in 1987, **The Omnibus Budget Reconciliation Act (OBRA)** or **The Nursing Home Reform Act** was passed by Congress to provide guidelines for the operation of Nursing Homes. The magnitude of these instructions has been overwhelming to most facilities. Individual States have challenged the Federal Government about many of the requirements and only now are they being enforced. **Most of our current procedures in Nursing Homes are the result of OBRA regulations.**

problems of the Administrator

All the problems of the DON are problems for the Administrator. He must also be a sounding board for the staff. He must instill group purpose and establish the goals.

Although Nursing Home law has been around for some time, the complex relationships of the staff, the Worker's Compensation procedures, grievance guidelines, OBRA, OSHA, and many other policy matters, are creating more legal questions and liability.

The attorney for the Administrator has become an important agent in Nursing Home operation. He advises about legal matters and, like insurance companies, insists that certain activities conform to rigid standards.

The many waves of new laws and directives are complicated and intertwined, coming from many agencies of Government, including the State Department of Health. These regulations pour over responsible Nursing Home staff members almost faster than they can be assimilated. The Administrator is constantly under pressure to comply.

other administrative staff

Administrative staff has grown to help carry the burden. It now includes Public Relations persons, Social Service workers, and many others. Since documentation is so important to inspectors, there is a lot to be written and accomplished by non-medical personnel. All this is meant to assure quality medical care for residents.

SUMMARY:

The Health Care Administrator represents the Owners or Board of Directors. When operational problems cannot be resolved through the usual channels, he has the final word.

OPTIONS:

- Meet the Administrator in case there comes a time you need to discuss some important matter.
- Consult him on problems beyond the scope of nursing or when you find the staff indifferent to your requests.
- Feedback is important to all the staff but especially the Administra tor.

Chapter 6

THE DOC

getting the orders straight

> Every treatment or patient activity requires medical approval by the attending physician. Let him know who you are and how you relate to the patient. If he can't laugh, fire him!

A century ago doctors rarely became involved in the care of the feeble elderly. What could they do? What should they do? That condition seemed not to be as much a medical problem as a reality of life.

Aging is still a frustrating process for today's medical profession, not so much the process itself, but the attendant problems of management.

In an age of wondrous discovery and brilliant technology, restoring good health is paramount. Like old cars in constant need of repair, the aging, ailing body rarely returns to robust good health. Each illness leaves a deeper scar.

Yet more and more tests and treatments can be given. More services can be sought as part of team care. Caught between cost control and optimum patient care, the Doc is pressured on all sides.

In keeping with developments in knowledge, medicine provides state-of-the-art methods to replace worn out parts. Lens implants, hearing aids, heart by-pass surgery, cardiac pacers, knee replacements—the list is endless in terms of medical advancements which prolong productivity and extend old age. Newer medicines are much more effective in controlling heart rhythms, aiding digestion, etc. They are also very costly.

Yet many physicians who deal with aging are not as impressed with the applications of science as they might be.

What might be described as a laissez faire attitude about longevity has evolved into aggressive frontiers of treatment, some without medical evidence of benefit. We are no longer content to let nature take its course. Physicians intercede for the benefit of the patient and most families follow their suggestions.

medical dilemmas

When treating Nursing Home patients, however, the process of decision making is even stickier. The risks are higher. Outcomes are less predictable. To make management matters worse, there is an over-the-shoulder scrutiny that rises from Government, lawyers, and outside interested parties. With the brilliant perspective of hindsight they know what should have and could have been done. Working within this sphere of activity has never been harder.

The Nursing Home Doc is the established authority, having been delegated the legal responsibility for his patient, as the current Nursing Home setting has become an extension of the hospital medical ward.

Not every doctor enjoys this particular role however, since he does not often feel in control and is often poorly appreciated for his interest. He frequently presides over a losing battle—one crisis after another for which a "good" solution is rarely possible. Trained to be a "hero," he seems often to be a "goat." Things usually get worse, and he's the mastermind of record. Younger doctors are often uneasy geriatricians. Understand his predicament and you may discover a "reluctant hero."

staff membership

Newer Federal regulations require all physicians to be approved for staff membership much like the detailed process that acute hospitals require. Before being allowed to treat patients, physicians must provide evidence of licensure, competence, training, malpractice insurance, etc. Once approved, he must agree to abide by the rules and regulations of the institution, and fulfill all his prescribed responsibilities.

duties and responsibilities

At the time of admission the doctor must certify the need for treatment, the expected length of treatment and stay, and render a prognosis; his expectation for recovery. If insurance applies, he must sign a "Certificate of Need" to authorize coverage for the condition.

Within 48 hours of admission, the attending physician must perform a complete physical examination on the patient, recording his findings on the record. Additionally, he must make a statement of the patient's awareness of his condition, note whether or not the patient has been informed and if not, why. Again he must prognosticate about what he expects to happen.

Every service to residents hinges on the "doctor's orders." In Nursing Homes they must be precisely written to spell out the medication and dose, the timing, the condition for which they are given, the expiration of the order, and if an "as needed" or "prn" schedule, what judgment should be used before dispensing.

Through the month he receives telephone calls about minor changes in condition, and signs orders mailed to him to be returned to the Nursing Home. He discusses over the telephone the resident's condition with family members or social workers or concerned nurses. Medicare expects all of this to be **quality care** and yet authorizes the physician to see the resident no more than once monthly.

For an emergency visit, Medicare will require a written explanation of services. Seeing two patients in the same home on one visit will result in the second fee being cut approximately in half.

He is expected to order laboratory tests on a periodic basis for patients on long-term medicines, such as digitalis, thyroid or potassium-reducing drugs, to insure that treatments are working effectively and without side effects. For many years these drugs were used without such frequent testing. He must explain and justify any deviation from protocol on the patient's record.

Either he or a colleague must be available for emergencies around the clock, 24-hours per day.

Any treatments given must be evaluated periodically, recorded on the chart and the patient re-certified if necessary.

Complete physical examinations are required of all patients yearly.

At death, he or a qualified licensed nurse must officially pronounce the patient dead. He must order the release of the remains to a mortuary. Within a few days, he must write a Summary of the patient's course while in the facility.

Many physicians find all of these Nursing Home requirements to be too demanding and restrictive.

Humor

Humor is the essential ingredient in caring for the aged. Otherwise, Nursing Home life might be intolerable for everyone.

Finding joy in simple things, irony in the fates, happiness in some small discovery—all give zest to living and elevate it above the ordinary.

The white-coated, stiff-spined, fixed-faced, pompous practitioner that rises over the lowly, sprawled, thin, helpless figure half exposed by wrinkled sheets, is the specter of the godly healer. Unwilling to touch, requiring him to wash his hands, he sanctifies everyone else's presence. Such a doctor has no place in a Nursing Home!

Stooping to touch, listening close to the whisper, shouting into the deaf ear to be heard, a twinkle in the eye—these are the markings of a good geriatric doctor. Communicative skills are separate from learning skills or keen academic observation. Patients need doctors with all of these.

The astute clinician and caring physician knows how to approach people, open a dialogue, read the body language of those around him. **Get one like that if you can find him or her!**

No one is perfect for each and every patient. Like our marriage partners or our friends, we all have our preferences. It's important to listen to our chemical urgings. Patients speak out not only verbally in the way they receive their respected physician.

Nowhere in the practice of medicine is the art of communication more critical—because it is so difficult! Residents are blind and deaf, sensory deprived, limited in expression, and slow and clumsy to respond. They need someone who understands that, someone who cares and will take time to solve the simplest problem—a sore toenail, the blaring TV of a neighbor, rough handling in bed, or a loose denture.

They need understanding, kindness, respect, and gentleness.

transmitting the feeling

I placed the physician third in the **Triangle of Care** because he is the least important if the others are effective. The Nursing Home and the family have more overall input in quality care. On the other hand his impact can be considerable where the others are not strong.

Doctors who **care** for their patients transmit their feelings to nurses, aides and everyone in the Home.

On the contrary, if they show disrespect or lack of concern, then why should anyone else worry? Concerned and giving people are essential in Nursing Homes, and thank heaven they seem always to be found. By their nature such people seek out those that need them most.

If a call from the Nursing Home to a doctor about a resident's welfare somehow creates anxiety or reproval over the phone, or disruption of the doctor's busy schedule produces negative vibrations, nurses who try to be responsible are degraded. They find their work distasteful. They will not continue to serve effectively, no matter how interested in their patients they may be.

Feelings are there to be felt by everyone. Anytime employees are made to feel stupid or foolhardy or are demeaned, they will look elsewhere for approval.

What might be said of Nursing Homes can also be said of hospitals or businesses or institutions of every kind. Happiness, warmth, concern, respect and appreciation are the essential glues that keep people together. **Doctors are key figures in a successfully-functioning nursing staff.**

Find a Doctor who is willing to bring all these intangibles into his work. Find someone who likes people and seems happy to be alive.

Find one with whom you can express your concerns and you will find *quality care* for your loved one.

A doctor who has known the patient and other family members or comes recommended by others will probably be a good choice. Having many similar kinds of patients is also likely to mean accessibility is good and interest is high.

Think carefully about what I've written and especially about the qualities you most admire in your own personal choice of doctor. Patients strive to be open and confidential with their physician. Occasionally they suffer through a relationship because they want a special expertise. That is a personal decision.

let him know

Leave notes for the doctor on the front of the chart. He will read them when he makes rounds. Note your telephone number and best time for calling, if that is necessary. Try to find a convenient time to talk or make an appointment with him in his office for such a purpose.

If possible, plan to be there when the doctor makes rounds to improve mutual understanding.

If you're not happy with the service, try to find better somewhere else.

Medical Director

To assist Administration in assuring **quality care**, the Government requires that every licensed Nursing Home have a Medical Director. Like a Chief of Staff at an acute hospital, he is responsible for overseeing medical activities of the attending staff. He reports to the facility Administrator any problem he finds. Among other things, he advises about medical protocol and reviews procedures, watches for evidence of infectious epidemics, and serves on the Quality Assurance Committee and the Utilization Review Committee.

Most Medical Directors are physicians who have several patients within the facility. The role he plays in the care of all patients is increasing in depth and complexity. Being available almost daily makes management of the day-to-day problems more effective. Many facilities suggest that patients choose him as their primary physician because of the continuity of care he provides.

Listed in **Appendix B** are the duties and responsibilities of the Medical Director relating to patient care. In certain situations he can help you where others seem unable. Feel comfortable about calling him whether or not he is your attending physician.

SUMMARY:

Interest in the patient by the attending physician is secondary in importance only to that of the family. He must function within a system of increasing regulation and meet new standards of care, often arbitrary. Appreciate his predicament and keep an open line to him.

OPTIONS:

- Every patient has the right to select a personal physician, provided he meets the standards of care required by Federal regulation.
- Find an physician who relates well to older patients and can enjoy them.
- All patients have the right to understand what's happening and what the condition and prognosis is. They can elect their treatment.
- Communicate with the attending physician. Short notes left on the chart or mailed to his office can be very helpful.
- When some aspect of care is unclear, if answers cannot be found elsewhere, discuss it with him.
- Ask for an update from time to time if care becomes long-term or takes an unusual turn. In acute situations you should not have to call but rather should be contacted.

Chapter 7

CONTRACTS AND SERVICES

what can be done?

> You contract with the Nursing Home to provide routine care. But, in addition, ready to provide necessary specialized treatments, an assortment of skillful professionals are standing in the wings waiting for the call to pitch in.

In today's world almost every relationship is reduced to contractual understanding. Before admission to a facility, either the patient or the guardian must agree to abide by the contract for services.

There is also an array of services available from professional providers who operate under contractual agreements with the Skilled Nursing Home or can be procured privately.

Every service to patients must be part of the plan of treatment prescribed by the attending physician. Some must meet the guidelines for Medicare reimbursement.

contracts of admission

Presented upon admission or shortly before is a host of fine-line typewritten documents. These often seem to come at a time of pressure when families want to get their loved ones in and are willing to sign complicated agreements without thoroughly understanding them.

Most of these documents are routine forms intended to facilitate the care of the patient. They are a necessary part of doing business and are meant to avoid entanglements. It is better to iron out questions before the fact than argue later. Consult an attorney if necessary.

I have listed the many documents included in the typical admissions package in **Appendix C**. Each institution has its own forms and conditions peculiar to its circumstances.

If possible, familiarize yourself with these forms before you face admission. Read the fine print carefully. Take a copy home for review. Most Nursing Homes will allow time for you to review them before signing. Feel comfortable to ask questions if you're unsure. Don't sign anything that is unclear.

important information

There is certain general information that will become part of the resident's record and you will be expected to provide the data close to the time of admission. They include:

Next of Kin
Emergency Care Information
Insurance Information
Mortuary Information
Tissue Organ Donor Information

Families are important in providing information for the **Minimum Data Set (MDS),** a new OBRA document to be completed within 14 days of admission. This is a comprehensive 10-page computerized form that assesses the resident's function. It includes a lot of historical detail useful in planning goals for the resident.

patient rights

A **Patient Bill of Rights** document will be given to you to inform you of the laws governing the patient and how they should be implemented within the facility. **Appendix D** is a simplified version of the current OBRA directives. It is required to be posted in every facility, outlining the protection that the laws provide for Nursing Home patients. Many more rights are implied in other Nursing Home requirements. This book will discuss almost all of these areas.

You may be surprised at the wide range of freedoms they provide. Implementation of all of these rights has not been easy for some Nursing Homes. As you visit frequently, you may find more questions later on than in the beginning.

advanced directives

The Patient Self-Determination Act of 1990 (see Appendix E), implemented in December 1991, not only requires that you be notified of **Patient Rights** but that you be offered the opportunity to sign **Advanced Directives** before admission. These include **The Durable Power of Attorney for Health Care and Directives to Physicians,** such as **The Living Will.** The right to accept or reject medical or surgical treatment is also provided for at this time. Since this Act applies to hospitals, HMO's, and other provider organizations as well, there will be many opportunities to consider these matters long before Nursing Home admission.

A newer aspect of Nursing Home care is the focus on emergency procedures and even more specific treatment requests while in the Nursing Home. These can be implemented later but come up for consideration upon admission. A good understanding of these issues is necessary. In **Appendix G** you will find written samples of these types of **Advanced Directives**. They include:

Emergency Life Support Services
Directive to Physicians Regarding Treatments
Directives Regarding Intensity of Care

I will discuss the entire issue of "**BODYRIGHTS**" which includes all types of **Advanced Directives in Chapter 22**. They are important instruments in guiding your doctor in the choice of life-support systems should the patient be rendered incapable of speaking for himself.

After you have finished reading ***OPTIONS*** you will find it easier to make a selection.

services

A. Health Care Providers

physicians
dentists
podiatrists

These services are privately arranged. Most facilities have contracted with all of these providers as back-up to those of record. All must conform to Government regulations in the management of patients.

B. Pharmacy

The pharmacist is an important consultant. He oversees the administration of medications. Each medicine must satisfy a diagnosis. Otherwise it is not given. Incompatibility and excessive use are monitored carefully. He sits on several patient care committees to advise about the proper use of pharmaceuticals.

The contracting pharmacy provides medication in the unit-dose system. Each dose is individually placed in a blister pack envelope to minimize errors. He also maintains an Emergency Medicine kit for use on the ward. The pharmacist is on call 24 hours each day to furnish drugs on a timely basis. His inspection of all medications brought in from outside pharmacies is meant to insure propriety. Most residents use the contracting pharmacy.

Although you have the choice of using your own pharmacist, he must comply with the requirements of the Government regarding packaging, delivery, etc. These are carefully regulated.

Bedside over-the-counter (OTC) drugs are considered a patient right if residents are competent to manage them. Most doctors object to drugs of any kind, even those in locked drawers, if they are within reach of confused residents.

C. Inhouse Providers

- Physical Therapy
- Occupational Therapy
- Speech Therapy
- Special Assistance
- Restorative Aide
- Private Duty
  - Companion
  - Aide
  - LVN
  - RN
- Social Services
- Administrative Assistance
- Beautician
- Activities Services
- Laundry Services
- Transportation

D. Others

- X-ray
- Laboratory
- Outside consultations
  - Visits to specialized areas
  - Ophthalmologists
  - Ear, Nose, and Throat specialists
- Bookkeeping Services
- Counseling
- Ombudsman

Most of these services are self-explanatory and can be discussed with your physician or the ward nurse.

Consultative services provided by contracting professionals are billed privately. The facility bills for those which are provided by their employees. Billing practices are in part controlled by Medicare.

the ombudsman

Everyone's overseer is the Ombudsman. An arm of the Government, he is available whenever problems arise that relate to an individual's rights, appropriateness of care, legal matters, or management. He has the authority to act on behalf of the resident at Government expense.

benefit versus risk

As with every medical decision, there is the weighty problem of expected benefit versus possible side effects or risks. These are not always easy to determine. Not all treatments are effective nor are they completely harmless. Costs are also important. These are matters to discuss directly with those involved.

SUMMARY:

There are many services available to patients if the attending physician requests them. Medicare and Medicaid may require certification and provide guidelines for use. If you are not sure about any of them, ask.

OPTIONS:

- Make yourself aware of all the choices you have before signing legal documents.
- Advanced Directives signed before admission will become part of the record.
- By law a resident cannot be discharged from a Nursing Home except for very specific reasons such as failure to pay or uncontrollable behavior.
- Do not take valuables into a Nursing Home. Unsecured diamond rings and jewelry are easily lost. Label your own clothes with permanent laundry markers.
- Study Patient Rights to satisfy yourself that they are being met.
- Ask for special services if you think they are needed. It may cost more, but ask!
- Do your best to see that the resident's wishes are followed on questions of life-support measures. The written directives should provide most of the answers.

Chapter 8

PAYING

The cost burden

> As the technology of caring moves into high gear, assets of a lifetime can erode very quickly. Whose burden will it be? Who can keep up?

With Medicare in 1965 came a new role for Government, providing medical care for those elderly eligible for Social Security. The Government found itself drawn, first into promising, and then into providing more and more benefits to a surprising crescendo of dependent citizens, of all ages.

Today 75% of Nursing Home costs, $300 Billion per year, is provided by the Government. Medical cost projections for the year 2020 are estimated at an astounding 37% of the Gross National Product. Today's costs were regarded as astounding estimates 25 years ago.

What once was such a simple setting has become an extension of sophisticated living, the focus of life-extending activities.

The resident may not wish such an elaborate setting but many regulations that once applied to hospitals are now applied to Nursing Homes. Costs are skyrocketing in both industries.

newer expenditures

Every aspect of Skilled Nursing Home care is steeped in regulations, inspections, and documentation. No longer are there simple formulas for care. Many requirements for meeting "standards of care" are actually requirements for more highly skilled workers. Workers at all levels currently require more training and more supervision.

The Nursing Home environment has become a kind of ecosystem; temperature and humidity controlled, infection monitored. Every service to patients is guided by a host of printed requirements, from the timeliness of the food service, the dispensing of medications, to the disposal of body fluids.

Applying the same standards to each private home in this country, would disqualify most of us from being part of modern America. The computer database information form ,**Minimum Data Set**, now required on admission will no doubt be expanded in the future to involve even more costly technology.

Translated into dollars, that means residents will continue to pay more for whatever they get and costs will rise even more dramatically.

Medicare A

If skilled nursing is required after hospitalization, Medicare A will provide insurance coverage for a number of days before the patient is returned to the previous setting. Depending on the circumstances of the illness, this can apply for **up to 100 days**. Usually, it is a matter of one or two weeks. After that, the patient pays or supplementary insurance applies.

Many patients do return to another level of care and escape long-term nursing. Those who need continuing care, considered to be custodial, provide for themselves, usually from private resources. Only a small percentage of Medicare A dollars applies to the operation of most Nursing Homes.

Thus begins the financial drain which depletes the great majority of residents of their assets.

average costs

Routine costs for Nursing Home care in this country run $2400 to $4000 per month. They are increasing daily.

Because of the way this payment eats away the average resident's assets, 75% eventually become Medicaid (Medi-Cal in California) patients, dependent on State and Federal monies.

Measuring the quality of treatment against the cost is difficult. There are many variations from coast-to-coast and considerable individual factors in the operation of a facility. Insurance company interpretation of qualification for Medicare differs widely, even in nearby communities.

for the money

Comparisons are always made to staying in a luxury hotel for a day or a week. The major difference is the cost of companions. In a Nursing Home there is someone to dress you, bathe you, serve food each meal, bring water, move you across the room each time you wish to have another view, moniter and administer medications, flush the toilet or more demanding, clean up after you. This kind of companionship is a twenty-four-hour day offering. Find a hotel with that service and ask the cost!

Trained professionals cost money, especially if they are required to supervise closely day and night. Registered Dieticians oversee the food and others record how much of each meal is eaten. A log is routinely written about daily events but particularly if something unusual happens.

Environmental tests are conducted at intervals to assure temperature and humidity control, air flow, filtration, etc.

Inspectors number by the dozens. Besides the Nursing Home staff and consultants, the fire inspector, insurance brokers, City inspectors, State inspectors, Federal Government regulators—all routinely make rounds to oversee the operation and report their findings. Higher up, they are reviewed again.

Under such circumstances how could the costs be more reasonable? You may make your evaluation, but today's rates are set. There can be no bargaining in the monthly charge.

extras

Insurance companies want detailed records of services and their actual costs. Nursing Homes, like hospitals, have unbundled services, i.e. charge separately for each and every item supplied as a matter of more accurate accounting.

For patients whose daily needs are unusual, those extra costs can mount quickly. Before admission, when looking at costs, you must consider "special needs." Dietary supplements, equipment rental, pharmaceuticals, laundry service, and special treatments can be very expensive. Frequent diapering alone can mean hundreds of dollars extra per month.

As with all businesses, some manage better than others. Profit is an important part of the free enterprise system.

insurance

Unfortunately, the cost of critical care medicine is astronomical in today's acute hospitals. Full insurance coverage is not affordable for most.

Once insurance is expended in the acute hospital, it has some part to play in the Nursing Home system, but not much.

Less than 2% of payments to Nursing Homes come from personal insurance plans.

Many benefits are predicated on Medicare approval, a fickle and ever-shrinking cloak.

The cost effectiveness of insurance has always been at the heart of this problem. Senior citizens find the premiums large for the paid-out benefits. Most never expect to use such insurance and for that reason find it easy to decline. As it applies to Nursing Homes, buying secondary insurance should be considered very carefully.

protecting assets

Protecting your "**BODYRIGHTS**" with **Advanced Directives** is one of the best ways to avoid financial ruin, which happens often if one survives a crippling illness by means of prolonged and intensive treatments (see **Chapter 22**).

Many books are written by today's attorneys which outline the ways to protect assets—to avoid paying them over to Nursing Homes. Spouses' assets were once depleted before some of today's legislation was enacted. There are still some legal loopholes which make it possible to avoid being rendered penniless before being eligible for Medicaid coverage.

It is not within the scope of this book to elaborate on these details. If you feel uneasy or threatened, get some legal assistance.

Nursing Homes are required to provide information to residents about eligibility for programs such as Medicaid before private funds are depleted.

the poor

As the aged are depleted of energy and productivity, they often are also depleted of accumulated assets. Even those who manage to stockpile reasonable assets for emergency use, can find themselves without resources to cover the expense of long-term Nursing Home care. Most residents, in fact, become poor and eventually rely on Government funding.

For those who are poor when they first need Nursing Home care, the choices can be slim. Usually only Medicaid homes are available. Private paying residents have always subsidized Medicaid care where there is a mix. But where there is only Medicaid, funding will not permit increased numbers of personnel. The ratio of staff to residents is lower. The care is less.

Patient Rights, however, are not different. The approach to getting quality care is not different either, although it may be more difficult to gain.

SUMMARY:

Measured against the cost of Nursing Homes, all other kinds of elder care are a pittance (excluding round-the-clock private duty nursing care). For that reason alone Nursing Homes are a last resort.

OPTIONS:

- Avoid a Nursing Home if something else will do.
- There are differences in cost. Shop around. Find out what is included in the monthly charge. At the time of admission, Nursing Homes are required to reveal those services which cost extra.
- Be honest but use all the resources that are legally available.
- Cost burdens have become a way of life. Most residents actually deplete their own assets and fall back on the Government. In today's world, lack of funds will not ordinarily change the course of one's life.
- Patients are not segregated or labeled on the basis of finances.
- Spouses' assets are partially protected. **At this time families are not financially liable.**
- Avoid being angry with those who operate Nursing Homes. They are not responsible for the financial atmosphere.

Chapter 9

ON THE FLOOR

all in a day's work

> If you missed boarding school as a youngster, you may yet learn what it was all about. Certainly, on a practical level, there are many similarities to group living of all kinds—military life, the college dorm or fraternity house, a boarding home, etc. In all, the wishes of one are subordinate to economy and the common good.

An integrated staff works together. They help one another. They are a team and should relate well to one another. In a good Nursing Home, they are happy and you can see it.

There is no way to manage 75-100 disabled patients, the average size of a Nursing Home, without good organization. That usually means routines and schedules.

Individual preferences most often come second to cost containment and the general good. Nevertheless, flexibility is essential to appropriate care.

breakfast

"Rise and shine," the usual wake up call, signals the beginning of the day. More often for the elderly, the morning light is the usual alarm and their eyes are already open. Sleep is never deep and dozing occurs most of the 24-hour-day. The morning call then is not often disruptive.

Inactive bodies are usually anxious to move about and begin something new. Breakfast is the universally accepted and favorite meal with lots of choices, from cold to hot. Food is a good incentive to "shake a leg." Every mealtime is an important occasion, appetite being one of the last drives to slow down.

The staff is oriented to getting everyone dressed and up to the dining room in fine fashion. They encourage residents to participate as much as they can in an effort to stimulate the senses and create muscle activity.

This meal is usually the primary nutritional source for the day. After breakfast, it is more often pick and choose, as the foods begin to vary, and appetite wanes through the day.

The chattering among the staff is reminiscent of family living where youngsters are always excited about what's going on. Although conversation may not involve them directly, residents identify with the speakers and vicariously enjoy the enthusiasm of the others. Most

Nursing Homes have a clown, someone who acts up to entertain the others. There are bit players as well. Usually the time is a happy one when all are together to enjoy a common interest in food, hopefully good and nutritious.

Gathering everyone around the table and serving the meal takes time. Meals are usually long and complicated because many patients need to be fed or at least partially assisted. Keeping the food hot is a bit more difficult. Vision, hearing and thinking impairments hinder the conversation. Some residents sleep before the meal begins or once it's over. For special reasons some receive their meals in bed, alone.

Dieticians make considerable effort to satisfy individual appetites. Because of very common GI disorders, Diverticulosis, Hiatus Hernias, etc., special diets are common. There is a great effort to vary the menu without disturbing its nutritional content. Curiously, many of the "allergies and intolerances" and distastes for certain foods fade as the sense of smell and taste decline.

mornings

Although some go back to bed to digest their food, morning activities begin after breakfast. These are usually posted on the daily bulletin board and are under the direction of the Activities Director, a very important member of the staff. Her efforts are directed toward improving resident self-esteem and confidence via activities and social interaction.

Most facilities try to provide many stimulating activities for their residents. The deaf or blind are drawn in close. Each one is accommodated as well as possible. Reading, music, and slide shows are frequent and popular. Arts and crafts are common. Many have their own agenda. Quiet or nap times are interspersed with programmed activities. Residents can decline if either interest or energy is lacking.

Sometime in the morning, showers or baths take place, usually two or three times weekly.

afternoons

Lunch signals the beginning of the afternoon when outside events and special trips occur and visitors often arrive. A nap is once again a quiet interlude.

dinner

The end of the active day comes with the dinner meal after which time residents more or less go their own way, except for very special occasions.

Through all of this, residents are herded about by the staff often in the spirit of a group picnic, a few restrained to prevent falling or tumbling out of the wheelchair.

restraints

We must not forget to cover the important issue of preventing injury and the use of "restraints." **Appendix F** provides a list of the usual policies and procedures used by Nursing Homes in regard to restraints. The word itself is rarely spoken or written. "Postural supports" sounds better.

A few residents are able to ambulate freely. But because of reduced strength, poor balance, confusion, as well as for other reasons, others can walk only with the steadying hand of a "restorative aide" or attendant. Families are usually welcome to participate in walking their loved one. Some residents cannot support their body weight and can never walk.

While sitting in a wheelchair the urge to reach out, stand up, walk to the bathroom, or help someone else is beyond recognition as a dangerous maneuver. **Restrictive devices that are used to prevent residents from taking risks are called restraints.**

There are many kinds of **physical restraints**, those used in a chair or wheelchair, those used in bed, those which prevent arm motion, leg motion, or body motion. Most are soft and safe.

When patients are being transferred from bed or wheelchair, onto the toilet for instance, temporarily unsupported, they can easily fall with attendants only inches away. The problem is one of constant surveillance and attentive assistance.

Incredible numbers of falls are encountered in Nursing Homes in spite of extreme precautionary measures. Some patients unwittingly untie themselves or others.

As a rule, patients become accustomed to restrictive devices and work around them. Regulations require that they be removed or residents be re-positioned frequently to prevent pressure sores, etc.

Unfortunately, those who cannot walk become special problems because of inactivity. Their bones become more brittle and breakable.

"**Restraint Free Care**" is the current effort to eliminate restraints of all kinds, a concept mandated by OBRA. The extent to which soft restraints can be removed is now under study. The Nursing Home industry is trying hard to provide care to the levels required for such care. This necessitates in-depth evaluation of each case and very close observation.

Family awareness of restraint policies will be necessary if changes are to be made. **Whether restraints are used or not, unwelcome incidents will continue to happen. It is the nature of Nursing Home life!**

drugs that calm

Where staff is not available to calm patients or manage various kinds of antisocial behavior, drugs have been used to lessen anxiety. Used in such a way, they become "**chemical restraints.**" Meant to modify behavior such as excessive anxiety, crying, hostile gestures, abusive behavior to others, depression, roaming, spitting, kicking, they also subdue physical activity. This reduces the risk of falls and at the same time the demand for nursing care.

There is a fine line between modifying behavior and reducing nursing demands which opens the way for criticism about the use of these agents.

The extreme case is the grossly delusional psychotic patient who is out of contact with reality, manageable only with antipsychotic drugs. Unmedicated, the patient is a danger to everyone. Few argue with such use.

But what about the little old lady who pushes or strikes others, a potentially dangerous act? Or the one who cries out again and again, an annoying but harmless act? How much medicine should we use in these cases?

Judicious use of tranquilizers sounds clever and artful but is never without the down side—namely, day-night reversal, shaking, rocking side-to-side, twitching, repetitive leg or arm motion, and drowsiness which sometimes permits the head to fall forward. No one more than the caretakers know how difficult that narrow line is to walk. It changes, too, just as people do, from moment-to-moment, day-to-day, and month-to-month and because of other medications.

abuse of restraints

Understaffed Nursing Homes rely on keeping residents subdued and restrained. They can do little else in order to manage.

Well-staffed and active programs use few physical restraints or restraining medications.

To avoid high costs of care, money managers and regulators find good medical reasons to restrict behavior-modifying medications. An agitated or abusive patient can wear out four sets of nurses' aids on one shift if simply accommodated or treated with a drug-free, hands-on approach. Not many caretakers could survive such day-and-night care giving.

For some patients there is no night—only a twilight that never unfolds. The use of sleeping pills or sleep aids is common in order to provide some rest for the central nervous system. I think they are helpful for many patients although their scientific usefulness has not been proven. Those that are not cleared from the body can act as daytime tranquilizers.

Many patients can do very well for a time without drugs. The idea of "**drug holidays**" has never been new. Results are often surprising and worthy of the extra effort. Very close observation is necessary when changes are made.

elderly abuse

Residents who cannot protect themselves or their assets are potentially subject to abuse. Long before the Nursing Home admission, the elderly are conned and cajoled by close associates, often family members. Though the laws of the land attempt to curb such exploitation, many kinds of abuse occur frequently, and go unrecognized.

Within some Nursing Homes we see patients treated as children, sometimes threatened or brow beaten, and occasionally physically mistreated by misinformed care givers. This is strictly forbidden and reportable to Government agencies. **There is no excuse for abuse of any kind!**

shifts

I mention the important fact that three shifts of employees are required to provide continuous 24 hour per day care. They are arranged usually 7-3, 3-11, and 11-7. Each shift has a distinctive function with quite different roles for staff members.

The personnel are different, too. You should know something about the full 24-hour day and would benefit by visiting at various times, but not as a habit.

SUMMARY:

Routines are part of the Nursing Home life. They become a life style and sometimes a rut. Every new excitement helps relieve the boredom.

OPTIONS:

- Learn the schedule of activities and try to fit in, contributing to other residents' enjoyment if possible.
- Understand the methods of restraining and be sure you understand why they are used for your resident. Review the policy with your doctor if you are unclear.
- Be sure you know what drugs are being used and why, especially if they are tranquilizers or sleeping pills.
- Good nutrition usually means a stable weight. As a general guide to well-being, watch the monthly weight chart. Sudden weight loss or gain is not normal or expected and must be routinely reported to the physician.
- Visit at odd hours to see how things are different and how your resident manages.

Chapter 10

OTHERS

fellow travelers

> Where patient care is good, usually there are many people around, especially in the daytime, including visitors.

One of the most difficult problems for residents is communicating with other residents. Friendships do not come easily.

For most of us the journey through life is not so much our own as it is those with whom we travel. It is our interaction with others that gives life meaning.

At first, it's our mother and father. Soon the rest of the family. Then our peers. We understand the world by watching them and choosing the things we want to do with them or for them.

Nursing Home travelers are a mixed bag of odd fellows (actually 75% women). Not that they can change or be accountable for what they have become, but the factors operative in early life are not functioning here.

There is no choice about the other residents. Like riding a commercial airplane, the available seat may be next to anyone. Free and easy companionship is gone. The closest relationships come mostly from care givers. Moreover, most residents have so many handicaps and/or confusion that the world shrinks about them to the immediate, severely restricting any intellectual pursuit except the simplest considerations.

private tables

Most tables are in fact very private. The sociability that makes eating so enjoyable through our lives can be reduced to a tray and server who may not have the time or interest in conversation.

More than 75% of Nursing Home residents have nervous or mental diseases which limit them. Vision and hearing are impaired in most. The other 25% have physical disabilities. All are experiencing general decline.

Almost everyone has a very close friend through most of a lifetime. But roommates in the Nursing Home, more often than not, may as well be in the next county. Although the staff attempts to create compatibility, it's more likely to be based on least disturbing or disruptive choices. The social amenities that we expect from others may not exist. Behavioral patterns that are antisocial and bothersome to others are common, sometimes resulting in patients being set-off from the others, segregated because of incompatibility—a policy that does not comply fully with the intent of patient rights.

Because many cannot see or hear, they have difficulty responding. The camaraderie that accompanies most group living is often sorely lacking no matter how hard the staff works to promote it.

daily reminders

More than anything else, the disabled are constantly reminded about age and debility and disease merely by being there. A sea of helpless old people surrounds them.

Sorely missing is the laughter of children and young people, the sounds that keep greying heads interested in living. When a local kindergarten comes to visit, smiles and excitement flood a Nursing Home as at no other time. Pets and animals bring on the same kind of joy.

Withdrawal, isolation, contentment with secret thoughts and feelings, these are the patterns we see in Nursing Homes. Blocking out confusion, denying the limits that aging imposes, the mind retreats to its quietude.

visitors

The strongest connection with the past is memory. The memories that family and friends bring inside a Nursing Home lift the mind back in time once again, whether to happiness or sadness. Nevertheless, deep recesses that lie dormant are reopened. Family and friends do that for all of us, recreate the past, sound out the present and imagine the future.

The intended role of the visitor has never changed. His presence is a light, a sign of allegiance, a beautiful memento, a voice from the past, a fulfillment of the desire to see the life of another as a means of understanding our own.

A pleasant surprise, a sweet treat, the gift of friendship, an inquiry, a touch, a foot rub, a song, a picture, a sound, a likeness to another, a contact with the living world—these are the things that a welcome visitor brings.

To the contrary, a condemnation, a reminder of stress elsewhere, an unhappy tone, a story of dissatisfaction, complaints directed at others, tears, anxiety, threats, browbeating, revenge—these are gifts from Hell. They have no place in a Nursing Home.

gifts worth bringing

As a visitor you are reminded to leave your tensions and anxieties at home.

Everyone feels it when a warm person walks into the room. He can light it up with expression, color, sound, harmonic interaction, kind words and gestures. No different than life on the outside, seeing family and friends is a natural high.

Bring happy memories. Recalling sadness and unhappy times may depress residents. If they must come to mind, end on a happy note!

Find points of interest from the past or recent excitement. Probe the mind of the resident. Discover the uniqueness there. Dwell on mystery, changes, new ideas, current events. The imagination is a wondrous escape.

Touch and show affection. Hugging and kissing are wonderfully healing expressions. Holding hands while talking helps concentration. Be excited about what you see. Try not to prejudge but look to understand.

Wear colorful clothes, bring flowers, smile and be happy. It's contagious. Open windows, introduce your own warm spirit. Find something to laugh about.

Be optimistic about the immediate future. To remind the resident of how little time is left or of unreached goals or impossible dreams is counter-productive. Try not to show discontent. If something is wrong, work to fix it.

Mention your next visit if it is soon. Leave them with a chuckle or laugh or an expectation of something exciting.

Remember to relate to others nearby. It helps everyone feel closer and a part. Become part of the esprit de corps.

If you feel rotten, stay home. Residents don't need cold viruses or other contagions in such close quarters.

SUMMARY:

The Nursing Home traveler is often alone. The needed companionship is not easily available. Every bit of communication, affection, attention, and love are wondrous events in a long and quiet day. Don't be afraid to give.

OPTIONS:

- Family and friends have free access to Nursing Home residents.
- Visit often. Bring gifts worth bringing. Enjoy your visits.
- Residents must be informed about roommate changes by the Nursing Home staff before they occur, except in emergencies.
- Show interest in other residents and their families. Friendship and kindness are much needed.

Chapter 11

MEDICAL PROBLEMS

the usual list

> We are born with soft skin and tiny toes. And each phase of life, each process of living endows us with new characteristics. Eventually worldly experiences mature and ripen us. Having been exposed to more or less the same things, in the end our tissues have many common features.

Reaching old age means having been through a wearing-out process. There are dozens of medical disorders that can be found on every patient merely because of aging.

They occur naturally and are common, very common—coming on, more or less, at the same time. Like puberty or menopause, they happen and leave their mark. Understanding the changing body leads to easier acceptance of the process.

the disease of aging

When we can be honest enough with our intellectual selves, we will call aging a disease. By almost any definition it is deterioration associated with chronic symptomatic disorders of most body components. Eighty percent of those over 65 have one or more chronic diseases. Ninety-five percent of those over 65 have some form of cataracts, for example.

Some professionals insist that aging is not a disease. Nonsense! **Aging is a disease of diseases.** Denying this truth is one reason that some have so much difficulty accepting the aging process.

Practically speaking, there is no such thing as "normal aging." The only question is at what point after sexual maturity does aging begin. Certainly, the onset of a chronic symptomatic disorder for which there is no cure, only palliation, seems the logical place. And that, for most of us, begins after 60, most surely before 65 years of age. It is the first crack in the armor we call health. The exceptional few who seem to manage robust living into advanced age are rare. **Nursing Home residents on average are in the advanced stages of aging.**

to begin with

Let's look at what almost everyone who reaches a Nursing Home will surely have experienced. I don't mean to characterize anyone in particular but refer to everyone in general. There are always exceptions, especially in degrees of involvement. And in truth, as men and women's genetic features are distilled through life's experiences, their characteristics and their scars are very unique and individual. They indeed become "characters."

This list is not meant to disturb the reader. It is the way things are and therefore needs to be appreciated if we are to understand the medical aspects of Nursing Home life.

There are only a few generalizations that are worth mentioning:

Women outnumber men three to one.

Fat patients are rare although mild overweight is common.

Smokers and drinkers and drug abusers rarely reach old age.

Fatigue and lack of energy are the most common non-specific complaints.

SKIN

The skin is dry and thin. It tears and bruises easily, especially in women. Small cancers can be growing among the aging spots, keratoses, and warts—the "barnacles" of age.

HAIR

Scalp hair is usually thin and sparse, permitting heat to exit the body more easily, leaving the patient cold. If there is little body fat, it can contribute to insomnia. A ski cap and stockings can be very helpful at bedtime.

EYES

Sharp near vision disappears in the 40's when glasses are needed for reading. Cataracts develop in the early retirement years. A score of other eye diseases related to blood vessel hardening or circulatory impairment are frequent. Muscles become weak around the eyes, permitting the upper lids to droop, the lower lids to fall out, hairs to turn in, and infection to develop.

Properly fitted glasses are an important tool of communication in the sensory impaired.

EARS

Hearing is diminished. Aids are often needed but are not often worn by those who lose more hearing after admission. Wax build-up needs watching. Episodic dizziness or vertigo is common, and tinnitus or ringing in the ears is very common.

NOSE

The acute sense of smell and taste is lost slowly, beginning early in life. Thin irritable membranes are common. Pollen allergies are less common.

MOUTH

Tastes are less distinct. Gums shrink as our teeth decay and are lost. Dentures get loose which may affect eating and nutrition. Like other portable appliances, they are easily lost.

NECK

Usually thin and wrinkled, the skin of the neck is likely to sag. The thyroid gland becomes smaller like most glands in the body.

BREASTS

The mammary glands are usually flat and less glandular. Having had tumors removed, many breasts have scars or are absent. Cancerous tumors continue to occur.

LUNGS

Chest expansion is poor. The spine collapses forward causing the shoulders to hunch.

HEART

Small collections of fat and cholesterol have formed in vessels all over the body but are more critical in the heart. Many have had slight injury, or muscle damage, often silent. Angina, or inadequate blood flow to the heart muscle, can be silent as well. These things disturb the electrical impulse (measured in an EKG) which is seldom normal, causing the heart beat to be irregular and prone to distressing rhythms.

ABDOMEN

Because of weak muscles, the abdomen is protuberant and may have scars of previous surgery. Occasional hernias can be found, sometimes in the scars.

GENITALS

Male: the testicles are small with sparse pubic hair. Problems with urination are common because of an enlarging prostate gland which sits below the bladder, thus restricting the urinary outflow tract. Many have had surgery to permit easy flow of urine. Microscopic cancers develop in men with higher frequency as they grow older. Cancers in younger men are deadly. They are less vicious with age.

Female: The pubic hair is sparse. Membranes are dry and thin and prone to irritation. Muscles are weak and leaking urine is common, but this is usually slight and manageable. The internal organs (if still present) are small. Cancer of the uterus, cervix, or ovaries can occur.

SEXUALITY

This aspect of behavior changes throughout our lives and is not limited to the sexual act. Both desire and performance decline after both male and female menopause, for some to vanish completely and for others to take on other aspects of conjugation. Vigorous and active orgasmic sexual activity in the advanced elderly is only youthful fantasy, a statistical rarity.

BONES

The joints are knobby from wear-and-tear arthritis, but motion is minimally restricted. Frank pain is uncommon but aching and soreness are usual. The spine loses its flexibility and strength. Bone structure becomes brittle.

BRAIN FUNCTION

Most brain function begins to decline measurably at about fifty years of age, fortunately very slowly. Other characteristics include slower thinking, forgetfulness, poor balance, muscle tremors, diminished reasoning power, and dozing through the day. Deep restful sleep is lost. Patients tend to fix on ideas, especially those of the past, and persist in talking about them. Emotions are easily upset.

INTERNALLY

The stomach slips into the chest (hiatus hernia) as the diaphragm muscle weakens. Gas and indigestion are common.

Pockets (diverticuli) form in the large intestinewhich sometimes cause a change in stool pattern and occasionally require a diet without nuts, seeds, skins or leafy green vegetables but still high in fiber. Psylium husks become a daily elixir.

individual differences

I've presented the substantive changes of old age to which must be added the very individual experiences which make us all different. Now that you see how the whole system is affected, you will appreciate how new problems might occur atop the others.

The best protections from early aging are inheriting healthy genes and continuous activity, both physical and mental. Actual tissue growth can still take place with exercise, even in old age. Many robust older patients demonstrate the value of active minds and bodies.

Ailments

In order of frequency, the following are the most common ailments that afflict the elderly in a Nursing Home. **For many they are the precipitating reasons for being there.**

SKIN TEARS

As the skin grows thin and loses its elasticity, it tears like tissue paper, with even the slightest pulling. The longer we live, the easier we tear. This is the most common injury in a Nursing Home and is often an indication of the longevity of its patients rather than an indicator of careless handling, which, of course, it can also represent.

INCONTINENCE

Weakness of the muscles is never more embarrassing than when the bladder or rectum loses control of its contents. Incidental bacterial invasion of the bladder is often present in women. Unfortunately, medications used for adding more muscle tone or antibiotics for the incidental invaders are not very helpful. The use of bladder training techniques, and external catheters in men are preferable to internal catheters. But all, like diapering, are costly.

CONFUSION AND WANDERING

There are many kinds of confusion. Some patients are relatively clear-minded at one time and confused at others. Most confusion is not harmful. Eating someone else's food, taking vitamins from another's nightstand, climbing into bed with an unsuspecting roommate—all can be problematic. Attending personnel usually manage these actions without difficulty.

Combine confusion with the urge to be active, and wandering away from the premises can be a serious matter. Patients can get to dangerous streets or other hazards before they are missed. Newer perimeter alarm systems are helping keep track of such cases. Restraints have been discussed in **Chapter 9**.

DEAFNESS AND BLINDNESS

These have been mentioned. Serious impairment of either organ can cause severe disability. It is important to keep hearing aids and glasses in working order. Their importance is often discounted after admission.

FALLS AND FRACTURES

You might wonder how so many falls occur in such a controlled setting, especially when restraints are so commonly used to prevent them. Weakness, poor balance, and faulty judgment, combined with a rare moment alone, will permit accidents to happen. Brittle bones snap easily.

Unfortunately, as is the case with fractured hips, if untreated surgically, serious nursing problems develop from immobility and pain. **More than 50% of hip fracture cases are dead within one year** in spite of intensive treatment. The fracture then may be but another indication of the extent of overall deterioration.

HEART ATTACKS

Lacking the usual sensory awareness, residents can have minor heart attacks, suffering damage to the heart muscle, without showing many symptoms. Sudden death occurs rarely.

SMALL STROKES

Small sections of the brain can have their blood supply cut off temporarily causing **Transient Ischemic Attacks (TIA's)**. Permanent damage is called a **Stroke**. The results are mental changes, behavioral changes, muscle weakness, or sensory impairment. These often produce slow decline with prolonged invalidism.

DEMENTIA

This will be discussed in more detail in the next chapter on Alzheimer's Disease.

PAIN

Pain is not a common problem. It is sometimes seen in terminal cancer cases where it can be controlled. Something serious is usually happening when a patient complains of pain. If simple medication does not relieve it, look for something of significance or unrecognized injury.

DEPRESSION

There are depression syndromes that can affect any age, even the very elderly. They usually respond to small doses of medication. In the elderly, more often they represent significant disease processes within the brain.

TEMPORARY ILLNESS

Colds, sore throats and stomach flus that exist in the outside world will generally find their way into Nursing Homes. They can trip a delicate balance. Most residents recover as they always have if complications do not develop.

DRUG REACTIONS

Most adverse drug reactions occur in the elderly at the time of life when most medicines are being used. They are usually manifested by rashes or stomach or bowel disorders. The old adage applies here: "Start low and go slow."

ABUSE

This has been discussed along with restraints in **Chapter 9. There is no excuse for patient abuse of any kind.**

UNUSUAL SIGNS AND SYMPTOMS

The typical complaints that accompany the beginning of a disease process, appendicitis for example, are often muted and confusing, even for experienced physicians. Missing in the elderly are the brisk responses, awareness of subtle pain, and changes in white blood cells that show infection. An acute abdomen or pneumonia may not be recognized until the process is quite advanced. These things make medical care even more difficult.

carrying on

Life is precious—one experience at a time. If only to have one more day—to see the sun rise—to look once more at an old photograph—to taste pancakes, syrup and sausage—only one event and nothing more, would anyone choose to live it through again? In my opinion most would say yes! Even though yesterday was about the same! Those with small kingdoms have simple wants. Some patients seem to want to last through the night, for just one more day. Others want to hold on and see just one more Springtime.

SUMMARY:

All body tissues experience the wearing-down process as we age. We are all exposed to similar agents resulting in similar disorders. In order to fully understand the disabled person, you must be aware of these many processes that are taking place simultaneously. They influence the way one thinks and behaves. They influence the ways one can be treated.

OPTIONS:

- Expect the aging process to continue and new cracks in the armor of health to develop.
- Recognize the difficult management problems of those who try to give good care 24-hours each day.
- Look for abuse. You have the right to expect care that is free of abuse and arbitrary restraint.
- Ask questions if you don't understand a particular aspect of care.
- Grant residents the right to enjoy their pleasures, however simple.

Chapter 12

ALZHEIMER'S DISEASE

a special case

> Tangles in the brain! Everyone has them but for some they are overwhelming. No one knows why!

Practically every symptom in this book deals in some ways with Alzheimer's Disease which in so many ways is similar to other "dementias" and disturbances of aging. Because no specific treatment is available, the general approach is often the same.

dementia

This is a medical term which refers to "loss of the mind," its literal meaning. Although in broad terms it might be applied to the mentally ill, it is used today to connote actual brain damage. The result is confusion, loss of memory and measurably-diminished brain function of a chronic nature.

Acute confusional syndromes, or delirium, are usually the result of an acute illness such as a head injury or brain infection, both usually short-erm conditions. Technically, these are not dementia.

Many diseases can cause chronic dementia including large and small strokes (localized areas of brain damage due to blood vessel disease), and chronic damage, due to infection, tumors, and injuries to the brain, etc.

Alzheimer's Disease causes dementia by interfering with function as **small "tangles" develop throughout the brain**. Normal aging brains have similar tangles, but very few. Alzheimer's Disease patients are riddled with this lesion, the cause of which is still unknown.

Described in 1907 by Alois Alzheimer, a German physician, it was once thought to be a pre-senile disorder, i.e. occurring long before old age. Actually it is found anytime after middle age, but is more prevalent in aged men.

Distinguished by its wide involvement of the central nervous system, it impairs function in almost every facet of brain activity. However, muscle strength is remarkably preserved until the later stages of the disease.

the differences

Alzheimer's Disease is progressive. The rapid form causes death within 3-4 years. On average, the course is about 7 years, but sometimes as long as 15 years after the onset of symptoms.

Latter stages require total bed care and are characterized by severe speech impairment, sensory and motor deficits, malnutrition, aspiration of food into the lungs, pneumonia, kidney infections, wasting and death.

Although newer brain scanning and imaging techniques can correlate at times with the clinical course to suggest the diagnosis, the definitive diagnosis is made only after death, at autopsy.

similar syndromes

In the beginning other kinds of diseases can, unfortunately, act in similar ways or may even accompany Alzheimer's Disease, thus clouding the diagnosis for some time.

Multi-infarctional dementia is caused by many small strokes. **Major strokes** can usually be identified as such. The early symptoms of **Brain Tumors** can be very deceptive for a long time.

Depression, thyroid deficiency, and other diseases cause similar signs and symptoms but can be helped with medication.

Drug reactions may suggest Alzheimer's Disease but symptoms clear up when medication is discontinued.

Parkinson's Disease is very different. With its characteristic pill-rolling tremor, rigid muscles, shuffling gait, drooling, tiny writing, etc., it is not one of the confusing cousins.

Before today's highly-detailed brain scans, many of these diseases were lumped together and treated similarly.

a common occurrence

Alzheimer's Disease has become so common that it is said to account for 40% of admission to Nursing Homes. What features distinguish it from the others are its usually progressive and dramatic downhill course. The disruption of activities of ordinary living are indeed profound. The intensity of care required is greater than the rest, often calling for closed wards, greater amounts of medication and increased use of restraints.

fears of inheritance or chemical exposure

There is no conclusive evidence of genetic transmission or communicability of one to another. However, new evidence suggests that there may be some genetic factor in the Alzheimer's Disease that occurs in younger patients, those under 60 years, where the occurrence is equal among men and women.

No specific chemicals, or exposures, or occupational hazards are recognized. Most believe the increased incidence is strictly based on the numbers of patients who are living longer. Some concede there could be a true increase in incidence due to some as yet unrecognized factor.

treatments

Understanding this condition has not been easy. Many studies are being conducted to find drugs that might help.

No practical or helpful medicines or therapies, including psychotherapy, are known. Some mood-altering drugs can ease the stresses and affect behavior, making nursing care a bit easier.

Quackery thrives in circumstances where there are no proven methods. **Choose wisely when you want "too desperately" to find help.**

taking the blame

Of all the conditions which evoke guilt or blame on the family, Alzheimer's Disease has the greatest potential. Clearly the process is actual brain damage. Yet spouses are often made to feel inadequate. They are easily caught up in a "guilt trip."

If you choose to blame yourself for what happens to others, you can find much grief and anguish here. Overly possessive or overly dependent personalities can find themselves in the middle of every threat, accusation, accident, setback or pain. Those spouses who are not willing to "let go" provide care givers with two patients—not one. Frustration abounds for everyone.

If you think of Alzheimer's Disease patients as crossing a line of accessibility, a point of no return, and you can face up to reality by accepting that truth, you can cope. Time will heal the loss. Let it begin early, not after months or years of self-punishment. If you are a religious person, then look to your God and your beliefs for help.

Letting go! The secret is letting go! Be content to do your duty as you see it, without taking personal responsibility for all the things that will surely go wrong.

These are the things I discuss with my families as we face the dilemmas of "caring." These are the issues I had to address when I became a physician and found myself in the midst of very personal tragedies within the families who looked to me for help. It is easy to feel partly to blame. **Many other diseases can affect us the same way and should be dealt with similarly**.

specialized centers

More and more Nursing Homes will specialize in Alzheimer's Disease treatment. Because of the severity of the problems and the need for more one-on-one care, the costs will be greater.

SUMMARY:

Of all Nursing Home disorders, Alzheimer's Disease is surely one of the most disruptive—for patients, families, friends, and health care providers. Problems occur at every juncture, usually get worse, and financially can be ruinous. Don't cope alone! Get help from others. Accept and "Let go," early!

OPTIONS:

- If the diagnosis is not clear, avoid trying to decide whether or not Alzheimer's Disease is present. Medically speaking, labeling is not helpful unless it affects some other aspect of care or changes your insurance benefits.
- Get help for yourself when you feel the need.
- Don't stop expressing love even though it may not be well received or even understood.
- Avoid taking the disease personally or looking for your own failures. Be gentle on yourself so that you can remain strong.
- Take "vacations" when the pressure gets too much. Respite care is available.

Chapter 13

WHO CARES?

the role of the family

> What makes the world turn for residents is their ties with what went before. Family interest is the spark that keeps them going. A surrogate will do. Next in importance to the Nursing Home in the **triangle of patient care** is the family.

If ever one needs a guardian angel, it's when he relies on others for everyday needs. No one is more vulnerable to the whims of the system than those who cannot speak. Having an outsider who cares, communicates a special importance to the attending staff. It means, "Do a good job, I'm just as interested in this patient as you are."

Being loved or needed or wanted is reason enough to live. When all the other reasons are gone, love keeps patients going. They try to return affection. Because they feel needed, terminal cancer patients hang on in spite of pain.

If there's one key to quality care in a Nursing Home, it's the concern of family and friends. It's the reason you have chosen to read ***OPTIONS***. You want to know what to expect, what else might be done, and who is responsible to see that things get done. Because of your knowledge and concern, others will listen. Take on the role of ensuring good care and you will find it.

close family

Family life is the glue that keeps a personality together. The give and take, togetherness, oneness, chemical bonding, and love—they expand our inner selves. Like marriage, they add longevity.

Family ties are the strongest bonds we have in life.

The advanced elderly have lost almost everyone—their grandparents, parents, uncles and aunts, siblings, their childhood families, their closest friends, and in many cases their own children. They see those faces in their grandchildren, for some the only ones left to refresh old memories.

Family caring goes on. Moment-to-moment needs may be satisfied by others but the family offers assurance that the care is proper and befitting until the end.

adopted family

Sometimes distant relatives or friends, or merely someone who happens upon a patient in need, comes to the rescue. They provide some semblance of family, fulfilling obligations. They adopt a resident. Rather than "adopting highways," I think we should find ways to adopt the unattached elderly. This would be true kindness and caring because it would be without any public recognition or praise.

signs of caring

It is the visits, the conversation, the joy rides, the holiday cheer, that fill the void.

Unfortunately, residents cannot always respond appropriately and sometimes can seem unappreciative. I suspect that the influences are still felt and are beneficial, nevertheless.

those that are lost

When abandoned to disinterested parties, Nursing Home care becomes a matter of institutional policy. It rests on the shoulders of health care providers.

Government overseers are swamped with many demands. Sheer numbers of problems make frequent and personal attention impossible, regardless of the intention of dedicated Ombudsmen.

SUMMARY:

A Nursing Home resident without a strong family member or advocate can feel alone and forgotten. Interested family can make all the difference in the treatment received. Be active, supportive of the staff, and don't be satisfied until the care received is what you want it to be.

OPTIONS:

- Keep family life active for the residents.
- Visit often to give your share of support.
- Don't be put off by the lack of communication. Find your reward in giving of your time and energy.
- Adopt an "abandoned" resident, one without family, if you have the time, energy, and interest.

Chapter 14

PLEASURES

happy times!

> Without laughter or song or words to express feelings, how can we measure the joy in life?

For those who are active and energetic, it is hard to imagine pleasure in a wheelchair existence. Yet, those who are candid about their lives know how often they see things differently as they age. Indeed, life is simplest when we are young because we recognize so few options.

the use of time

If we see an infant fast asleep in his mother's arms as she rides a crowded bus that is full of people, color and excitement, we might conclude that the poor baby is missing out on something. Most would accept the idea that the baby needs its rest. On the other hand, to see an old-timer dozing in a chair and suggest that it is a waste of time or misuse of human creativity is to deny the kinds of needs that fill an elderly mind. Why not accept both behaviors as part of the characteristic stages of life?

when is happy?

Thinking we can measure the joy in life for one who may not be able to laugh or sing is at the heart of judgment decisions. We tend to compare others to ourselves, our own ambitions and feelings. When we can rule against the existence of an old worn-out body, declare it purposeless or pitiful, our own prejudices are showing.

The young look for physical activity as a measure of happiness. For those who can no longer perform, the mental side of life may be their principal source of pleasure.

respect

I rather think that **old age is**! It happens. Most who have experienced it are surprised at finding themselves "old." It is a shock, having seemed to come upon them so quickly.

Nevertheless, it needs the same respect we give to other phases of our life. It needs understanding and tolerance.

the senses

Whatever perceptions are available—light, sound, smell, touch, taste—are able to rekindle other similar experiences. Are they better the next time around? Can they be embellished?

time

Time clicks are certainly different as we move through life. If each new and exciting event is a click, then they seem to come at different intervals as we age. In the infant they seem slow, since they sleep so much and seem to do so little, hardly aware of what is happening, while processing a great load of new information. Adolescence finds the pace quickening. The late teens click away at a wildly fast pace, carrying over into the twenties and thirties. Then the clicks begin to occur farther and farther apart, especially after menopause, until in later years only a few seem to be heard.

Drifting time, almost timeless time. No wonder we who are active and independent find it so hard to relate to the handicapped elderly. But for them it is still moving and still clicking. We should be more understanding of this process and more accepting of nature's way.

appetite

Certainly one of the easy measures of interest in living is appetite for food. It is the last interest to fade. Watch the way food disappears from the plate or how favorite tasty treats are devoured. There is zest for living shown here.

the electronic expander

It's hard to gauge how much the electronic worlds of radio and television and now computers have expanded the capabilities of the mind. With sight and sound we have fostered greater understanding and meaning, provided more information in exciting new ways. For invalids these effects are even more dramatic, especially in the absence of other stimulating activities.

exercise

What is there about stretching our arms or back or, better yet, pulling on a bright new sweater? Motion is a wonderful accomplishment.

When one person touches another with warm hands, kisses the cheek, hugs, combs the hair or massages the back, what happens to each in the exchange? Why does man's blood pressure drop when he caresses an animal? There are chemical events occurring here that add meaning to life.

a twinkle or a smile?

As a physician, my principle role is to bring a sense of assurance to the patient. Assurance that I am really interested, that I am doing everything I can, that I acknowledge and appreciate the cooperation I receive.

With a bit of humor, I can lessen the apprehension about a medical problem, dissipate a worry. By so doing, I have done much to improve a healthy disposition. To activate the mind, release the wit and humor within, to evoke an understanding smile, to recall a story, to resurrect an idea, to prompt a belly laugh—all of these serve to relieve pain and brighten the day where medicines fail.

SUMMARY:

Pleasure does exist in an Nursing Home. It is not hard to find even though it may be a much rarer event than at other times of life. Placing a value judgment on it may be more than we have a right to do. For the rest of us it is probably more important to add to it, however small our contribution.

OPTIONS:

- Contribute to sensory awareness.
- Exercise the patient, body and mind.
- Bring the gift of laughter.
- Respect resident's perceptions and wishes.

Chapter 15

RELIGION

faith in their world

> Faith in God, faith in a creed, or faith in some person each requires faith in oneself. Belief is therefore one of the most powerful motivating forces in our lives. It translates into self-confidence, determination, learning power, healing power, and staying power.

Faith is established early in life and is meant to carry us far.

As a doctor, I have marveled all of my medical life at the staying power of people. When everyone has given up, a patient often comes back from the edge of death.

Unseen forces move us. They give direction to our existence. They create the energy that gives purpose.

Preoccupation with the next world is common as this world loses its luster. But when brain cells shrink, religious fervor declines. Though indifference to abstract thinking sets in, ritual behavior may continue—bead rubbing, praying, meditating or reading the Bible. Their significance may be hard to assess.

Learning how to deal with life's vagaries, changing cycles, and especially one's own death, are the foundations of most religious experience. Patients who have steadfast belief systems are indomitable—usually cheerfully accepting the path that looms ahead, however foreboding.

reinforcement

Reinforcement of belief systems is very important to many residents. Of course, it's a very individual matter.

Most institutions provide religious services for those who desire them. They want to provide residents with every possible means of communication and expression. Transportation to a place of worship by the family is usually welcomed in the weekly agenda, if not too demanding an exercise.

Prayers of any kind are pacifying and relaxing. When the eyes close, sleep may ensue as well. That can happen to anyone.

Families should feel free to carry on their religious habits as long as possible. Important rites can be conducted upon request. Priests, Rabbis and Pastors of all faiths are always welcome.

dealing with death

Most residents find their beliefs reassuring and calming. Most residents do not fear death. Early acceptance of death is very beneficial when the actual time comes.

SUMMARY:

Over a lifetime the mind accumulates a sense of self and the universe and an understanding of purpose. Though they may lose some intensity, these feelings carry us to the very end. Nursing Homes and families and doctors should respect the patient's beliefs whatever they are.

OPTIONS:

- The expression of religious belief is expressly provided for in the conduct of Nursing Home life.
- Reinforce the strong beliefs of a lifetime when they are needed most.

Chapter 16

EXPECTATIONS

the best possible outcome

> Never is the prospect for doing something more clearly understood than when there is very little time left to do it.

For the disabled elderly there are few things left to do. Most of their lifetime ambitions have been accomplished.

Their principal goal is to enjoy the last few days, free of pain, enjoy good food, find new friendships, reminisce about the past, and watch the world unfold its mysteries.

They wish to continue a lifestyle of activity as they are able.

what will happen next?

Families need to know what their family member wants and what might be expected to happen.

In the absence of an imminent threat to health, no resident really entertains the notion of dying in the Nursing Home. A healthy mind does not dwell on that thought. Everyone knows his time will come but few have an inkling of what to expect, what to look for.

Death without warning, **sudden death**, is actually rare although most anticipate it will happen to them.

As a prelude to death, **an acute illness** that overpowers the systems is much more common. I will discuss the problems associated with acute illness in the next chapter.

A "crisis" can occur which may invite hospitalization. This can mean successful treatment, of course, or can mean a long and difficult time in an intensive care unit. And it can also lead to death.

Fortunately, **a long and agonizing illness** is rare because of modern pain treatments and earlier withdrawal of life-support systems which most patients request.

With the advent of **"BODYRIGHTS"** legislation, many potentially long-term situations can be managed in keeping with the wishes of the resident, rather than at the discretion of the courts or squabbling families. **Chapter 22** will address the methods of insuring the patient's rights via the Durable Power of Attorney for Health Care, Living Wills and Health Care Directives. Worked out in advance by the patient, family and the doctor, they will be most helpful.

Occasionally a patient will change his mind in the advent of an acute pain or threatening condition. Whether pain or apprehension, or expectation of benefit, or confusion causes the desire for an ambulance or hospital, it is hard to know. Those situations must be dealt with as they develop. When a change of heart happens, it will frustrate those who thought they really knew what a resident wanted.

As systems fail, one by one, and faced with a recognizable danger, the mind realizes the inevitable is close and finally dispenses with denial. Even then there may persist the notion that although it's coming, it will not be today. The present is prolonged. Magical solutions can remain part of the thinking for some time.

the usual course

We should be looking for a safe passage, peaceful and comfortable final days, freedom from anxiety.

Most patients have a slow decline with diminishing function and awareness, actually with very little recognition of the acuteness of a new crisis.

Sudden changes do occur. They are common and expected by all who work there. Don't be surprised if doctors and nurses are not surprised along with you. They know how quickly situations can change and are not frightened. If things happen quickly, the course is usually shortened.

Actually most patients are not keenly aware of the process of dying, not nearly as much as those who watch and wait.

overrated

Dying is an overrated experience, I suspect. Most seem oblivious to their exit. In the long history of mankind very few seem to manage some memorable last utterance. **The conscious mind is not usually present at the end.**

For many, the precise moment of death appears to come as unexpectedly as birth. It has so little to do with the living process, the active creative life, it would seem to deserve less emphasis.

Death is the end result of Nursing Home life and everyone knows that. Although we speak of treatments and recovery and walking again and talking again, these are the little moment-to-moment psychological deceptions we use throughout our lives, employed to keep us bravely trying. Death is what we all expect to happen. Of course, it's no different outside of a Nursing Home, it just happens more often there.

I mention this thought not to make it a central issue of Nursing Home life, which it is not, but because no matter what happens as patients decline, nothing will change the eventual outcome. And that fact makes a difference in how we might approach problems along the way.

Nursing Home life is just one part of the life experience, one that many of us will come to know. Somewhere inherent in the living and dying process is some measure of quality, some measure of naturalism, some measure of individuality.

interventions

There can be meddling in the natural course of human existence. Scientific theories about nourishment, and prolongation of life can add to the choices about treatments. If and when changes occur in the medical condition, there are certainly many medical forces that can be brought to bear.

Patients and their families have options about many of these things. They should be free to ask questions and satisfy themselves about their wishes. No different than freedoms on the outside, **you can choose what you want to do.**

Pushing food or pouring water into a mouth is no guarantee of therapeutic benefit as benevolent as the intention may be. Choking and pneumonia and respiratory distress can be the expected and uncomfortable consequence. Forced feeding with tubes may do the same, as well as require restraints. Most patients are uncomfortable with a tube through the nose into the stomach.

Many of our treatments, however, satisfy the wishes of the observer rather than give substantive relief or support to the dying. The use of oxygen, intravenous fluids, and sometimes even pain medications, are ways of **doing something.**

SUMMARY:

Life teaches us to expect the unexpected. Actually I've found fewer surprises in Nursing Homes than elsewhere. Once patterns are established, some diseases have a very predictable course. Others do not.

OPTIONS:

- Decide what you think most likely will happen in order to prepare yourself mentally.
- Make your own choice of treatments. Act in the resident's behalf.
- Second opinions for surgery and other medical treatments may be helpful at times, and they are provided for by Medicare.
- Don't be surprised by sudden change!

Chapter 17

A CRISIS

sudden sickness

> A minor illness can be catastrophic if too many systems are already overburdened and barely functioning.

Although illnesses can begin abruptly, more often they have a subtle onset. Early manifestations are often insidious and deceptive. It is easy to fool the experts when the signs and symptoms are unusual.

The characteristics of acute emergencies—the sense of crisis that may accompany so many traumatic events of the young years, are not necessarily part of the crises of aging. A fiery will to survive, to overcome, is not often part of the equation. Replaced by resolve and understanding, great outward emotion is rarely expressed by the elderly. So many personal tragedies of all sorts have happened through a lifetime that personal upsets begin to be relatively less disturbing. If they are, it is often because they are worried about the reaction of those around them. To see an unruffled, relaxed and understanding attendant, be it a nurse or physician, tends to induce a similar attitude in the patient.

Families are often more upset than patients—and this emotion can be transferred back to patients, causing unnecessary agitation.

It's not easy to imagine that someone is quite comfortable with the notion of dying, and quite willing to submit to the universal force that returns each of us to what we once were. Yet many elderly patients accept that. They wish for an undisturbed tranquil passage—free of pain, free of emotions, free of tears, and free of interfering gestures from others. Patients want to know they are handling it well. **Never in life is reassurance a more important pacifier.**

Most want to look back over their lives with a sigh of accomplishment. Those who are satisfied with the past find contentment. When ideas have not been expressed, when wrongs have not been righted, when angry words linger or anxious thoughts dwell, peace of mind is not easy.

Those who witness the final hours need understanding too. They want to help provide a peaceful passage. By accepting the cycles of our lives as a part of the "genetic plan," they can make the most of each and every phase and accept the dying process.

the semi-emergency, a serious threat?

A sudden fall with bone swelling and pain is always a crisis. This is because of the nature of untreated fractures, which is to remain painful with motion. That will surely create nightmares in bed care. It leads to bed sores and bladder and bowel problems of all sorts. As with hip fractures for instance, they need emergency surgery, almost without exception.

The treatment of medical illness is a more difficult call. A slight difference in breathing can make a great difference in lung or heart function and circulation within the brain. Pain, fever, changing mental status, breathing difficulty—these are the worrisome signs of a serious medical problem.

Nurses are very aware of the patient's general condition and are quick to notify the physician of warning signs and symptoms. He must make the decision as to what steps need be taken next.

hidden conditions

As in any medical emergency there can be conditions that have not as yet surfaced. It may not be known until many laboratory tests and X-rays have been taken that such conditions exist. In the elderly any new problem can be a critical one.

Then comes the question of how much should be done to find out the extent of an illness and after that how much treatment should be given. These are not easy management issues. Everyone needs to pull together as a team in approaching the course of action. Having Advance Directives is especially helpful.

When directives are not clear and the family has dissenting members, the physician may have no recourse but to ask the court for direction.

life and death emergencies

Among the **Advanced Directives** listed in **Appendix G** are the options available to the family in case of an extreme emergency. These are signed on admission as I mentioned before. Each time something new happens these instructions are reviewed. Emergency choices might include:

- **Begin CPR and Call 911**
- **Hospitalize if necessary**
- **Treat in facility (do not transfer)**
- **No treatment**
- **Keep the patient comfortable**

These options are meant to give families time to make further decisions or reassess the situation. Only CPR takes effect at once.

CPR

Cardio-Pulmonary Resuscitation is the emergency treatment rendered to an acutely-unresponsive person, without pulse or respiration. The recognition that life-saving measures could be provided by lay persons with a minimum of medical training, signifies its importance in everyday living. Since the early days, of course, such training has been extended to thousands of interested persons and almost all medical personnel.

In emergency settings where young people are involved in some type of accident, a bystander could be dramatically effective in providing an airway, maintaining blood pressure with external cardiac massage, and rendering other useful first aid services.

When paramedics arrive with their special equipment, drugs may be injected, electric shocks may be applied to the heart and mechanical-device assistance may be given for breathing. These are administered under the direction of an Emergency Room doctor who is in radio contact. In the Emergency Room of a hospital to which these cases are transported, all means are used to preserve life, including blood transfusions, surgery, etc. Full hospital capability is exercised.

Unfortunately, not long ago broader applications were found, influenced in part by malpractice considerations. The practice of initiating CPR was unnecessarily extended to Nursing Homes and other inappropriate situations where a "natural death" was expected to occur.

Because CPR and 911 are so readily available, quick action is necessary. **Residents of a Nursing Home must elect not to have CPR or resuscitation will begin and 911 will be summoned.**

There is an important individual choice here that needs to be made. I've found that many misconstrue the full measure of CPR. It is only the first step of many which are meant to keep the patient alive. It is true that upon the instruction of a doctor the process can be stopped at any time, but most often there is no personal physician at hand for some time. The idea that only a few puffs of oxygen and a slap on the chest constitute CPR is not true, although physicians are personally free to exercise limited options.

Once the process is initiated, usually all measures are taken. Although patients are treated in Emergency Rooms and Intensive or Cardiac Care Units with ventilators and an assortment of complex treatments, **few survive, especially among the elderly**. Total costs can be staggering.

What might have been a quick and painless exit, the desire and anticipation of most, becomes an explosion of activity. This scene is often loud, frightening for many, including the patient. This is no longer simple Boy Scout resuscitation.

"**No Code**" is the term used on the chart to specify that no CPR is to be initiated. It is written on the orders and discussed in the progress notes by the attending physician. It is flagged on the front of the chart and verbally transmitted to the charge nurse.

A tag around the neck which says "Do Not Resuscitate," "No CPR" or "No Code" would do well to serve anyone who has already made this decision—especially in hospitals, medical centers, public places and other "high-risk" areas for resuscitation.

Unfortunately, some families are frightened by the idea of discussing CPR with the resident, feeling it is not healthful because of emotional trauma. **Unsettled, institutions have no choice but to initiate full CPR and make every effort to support the patient until full medical treatment takes over and continues in the hospital.**

backfiring

Taking the "do nothing" approach, we might assume that the resident's decline would be quiet and peaceful and rapid. Clinical knowledge might lead to that conclusion. Unfortunately, sometimes the patient lingers, defying all predictability. Everyone is at a loss to understand how or why some stay alive but they do. No one is happy about the actual clinical course. When a pacemaker or critical medication is withheld, the death that seems so inevitable does not follow. Sometimes not for a long, long time.

I say this to make the point that although at times we presume to know very much, we are humbled by reality. Doctors are not God and are subject to the same frailties as everyone else. **Our best decisions can be very wrong.**

SUMMARY:

Sudden illness is a common occurrence in Nursing Homes. Families should prepare their minds for such things and anticipate their responses. It may not relieve all the associated distress but it will be very helpful for the patient to have made early written choices.

OPTIONS:

- Understand CPR and its ramifications. A decision will be requested.
- Remember the wishes of the resident. Avoid being critical.
- Try not to change direction in the middle of the stream.
- Don't second guess yourself or others. Looking backwards is never difficult.

Chapter 18

NEARING THE END

approaching the crossing

> Watching someone slip near death is too much like looking in a mirror.

Anticipation of a wonderful event is exciting long before it actually happens. Anticipation of death can be a horror for those who see it happening to a loved one.

Whatever the chemistry of bonding, breaking those ties causes physical pain. Losing a family member or close friend is like having your heart torn out. Experiencing that feeling early in life with the loss of a grandparent or childhood friend may lessen the trauma later on, but then the anitcipation may be worse. One day we will be able to look back and understand it better than at that dark moment. Our life goes on and we will laugh again.

preparation of the elderly

As patients age, most lose their fervor for living. They acknowledge their mortality and begin to find the possibility of living a very long time rather depressing. They prefer to think back instead of ahead as reminiscences are usually happy. Each deterioration reminds them of earlier vitality. Energy ebbs and the lust for living eases. In fact, many wish life was over and voice such ideas. Intellectually wishing to close the book, they seem to welcome the event.

Each close call with death, each serious illness provides opportunities to ponder the matter. When they survive, they often wonder why. They come to accept their helplessness. They resolve to die.

Occasionally there is unfinished business or some secret anxiety that keeps them on the edge for a long time. Unable to close a chapter of their book, their exit seems premature and unfulfilled.

As a physician, I try to find the source of anxieties so they might be eased. I assure patients that they are doing well, even as they struggle. The chemical changes that occur near death can confuse. They may not be aware of the rapid heartbeat and breathing as others are. I like to focus on things that are comforting, i.e. the lack of pain, a feeling of peace, the color of a flower, a picture on the wall. **Reassurance that things are going well is our most effective ministration.**

Those who can accept their death usually let faith be their guide.

They feel in control. It makes the process easier.

pain

Pain is an electrical nerve impulse that is sent to the brain by tissues that are injured, usually for the purpose of self-protection and avoidance of further injury.

This stimulus is strong for a time until the chemistry of pain is depleted. In chronic conditions of deterioration those chemicals are also depleted. Before the brain ceases to function, the cortex or consciousness area is less sensitive or even inactive.

Don't assume that the process of dying will be painful. Those who have described death via near-death experiences often tell us of the absence of pain. I have talked to many of those who are in extreme circumstances, expecting to hear them tell me how bad they feel or how much pain they have, only to have them respond that they feel fine.

In our modern world, medication should be used freely to prevent suffering. We may use more than we need but that seems safer and kinder. As with those who undergo surgery, the memory of critical events is not recorded in memory or conscious awareness. I have seen very few patients who actually seemed to suffer before dying.

SUMMARY:

As death nears there are considerations that can make it easier. Clearing the intellectual slate of unfinished business is important to some. Reassurance that those who are left behind can manage is important. Reassurance that the patient is handling it well is essential.

OPTIONS:

- Give the doctor and nurses support for using helpful medications
- Avoid the pitfalls of treatment with antibiotics or fluids or force feeding, if they seem to prolong suffering.
- Discontinue unimportant medications early.
- Accept the dying process. It is predestined.

Chapter 19

CROSSING OVER

from dust to dust

> For those who are gone the struggle is over. But for the living the mourning begins.

There is no option for death. It comes to all.

causes of death

For the record, every kind of death is possible in a Nursing Home. That large roof does not protect us from the same kinds of tragedies that occur in the outside world.

Accidental death from fire, earthquake, an explosion, suicide, murder—they all can and do happen. Of course, these are very rare.

Statistically, Nursing Homes patients die of aging and the diseases of aging. The average age for men is 81, for women 84. The event is expected and most everyone is usually aware of its coming.

being near

Arriving in this world, we have at least our mother there and in most cases expectant relatives, father, grandparents, and often a physician, or nurse, or all of them.

Departure rarely finds the same ensemble. For many reasons, death brings an aversion that even the closest find hard to overcome.

One can die alone. When the process is slow, few can fulfill the need to be at the bedside around the clock. Rarely can a family anticipate the time of occurrence so as to be present.

Someone present at the end, with a touch, seems the human thing to do. Whether the dying patient is conscious, semiconscious, or even unconscious, I think the presence of another is soothing and reassuring. Because the sense of hearing may well be the last to fail, say the things that come to mind, the words that sooth, the words that will help them go in peace.

the crossing

We now come to the most unique and private moments of a lifetime. Others who have ventured close to death have remembered their view.

What has been described variously as the last conscious incident of life is the perception of a long tunnel around which all else fades and a walk to the end as if moving toward a light. This may be perceived as rapid, or slow or timeless: minutes, days, weeks or years. These perceptions may not be framed in time spans as we know them.

Similarly, as we climb a mountain to behold the horizon, the miles of intimate detail along the ascending trail are lost in the magnificence of the distant view, beyond sight, beyond imagination.

I'm not sure that death is not akin to these or other similar experiences. But I've always been impressed by the indifference of the sojourner once the exodus begins. Those who have come back from near-death experiences, even though in pain or what seemed to be an agony of some kind, report a peace and tranquility, a certain pleasure in the process.

As observers, we should grant the gift of respect for those who cross over, their wish for comfort, pain relief, companionship, and religious absolution. I believe human beings have the right to approach that crossing as their faith tells them they should.

How a person died has none of the significance of how a person lived. The death act may be remembered for a time but the rest of the story is what is important. Few men are famous for their dying except in fiction.

when breathing stops

Although sudden death does occur, more often patients drift away in a sleep-like state, from consciousness to unconsciousness to coma, unresponsive to all stimulation. Breathing can be rapid and steady, more often it becomes irregular with long pauses. The pulse usually accelerates until near the end when it can become erratic and slow.

A last gasp or several may occur, sometimes minutes apart. That unique human being that has journeyed so far, finally quiets, and the crossing is complete.

feelings of loss

There are differences in the feelings we have about losing someone who is elderly from one who is young. There is a sense of completeness with the elderly, of fullfillment of all of life's cycles. Not so for the young where death seems so tragic and premature. In both cases, wherever there was some element of pain or discomfort near the end, there is a feeling of relief.

Expressing these emotions to fellow survivors is helpful for all who were near and dear. This permits them to close a physical relationship and begin an intellectual one built on memory. It brings them to an understanding of a kind of immortality that exists for all.

notification

An official pronouncement of death, certification that all life signs are gone, by someone licensed to make such an observation is necessary. Then notification of next-of-kin or responsible parties takes place.

The doctor must order the release of the remains to the local mortuary.

Personal effects are given to the responsible person.

The physician must write a Summary of the Nursing Home stay and complete the medical record.

SUMMARY:

Like life itself, dying is almost never without incident. Disturbing things can happen but they never seem to be noticed or remembered.

Our own concepts of dying will change as we observe it happen. We learn by watching others. In fact, that may be our only conscious death experience.

OPTIONS:

- Be present at the time of death if that seems right, but don't feel guilty if you cannot be there.
- Don't be frightened.
- Hold their hand if yours is strong.

Chapter 20

SETTLING UP

good-byes

> Say "thank you" to those who made the living easier for your loved one. These simple words are more important than gold to those who find friendship important.

There is one way for those who die to speak again, through their family, to those who were kind. Nothing can replace a personal gesture of appreciation from one to another.

unfinished business

Somewhere in the trappings of ceremony, very simple courtesy can get lost. Grief can disturb our actions, even simple acknowledgements.

Nonetheless, I have always been impressed with how many times a family will remember to send a thank-you note, flowers, candy, or some token of appreciation to the Nursing Home staff.

Unsaid, it can leave some doubt as to how well they performed a service. Good care deserves recognition. The substance of the gift is not as important as the gesture.

You should also let them know if there were any problems. A tactful suggestion is very welcome. That feedback is important to the staff. Most try to be very helpful.

turning to others

Many families will find other residents in need and will visit long after their family member has gone. This is another way to be appreciative.

Many families make the journey back to a Nursing Home to say good-bye and thank you, face-to-face with those who were caring.

SUMMARY:

Remember to show appreciation to the Nursing Home staff for their care. It bolsters morale and adds to the spirit of accomplishment. Many other patients will benefit.

OPTIONS:

- When the time is right, remember to say thank you.
- Go back and visit those whom you befriended.
- Gifts that help other residents are another nice way to say, " thank you."

Chapter 21

TOMORROW

for those who go on

A wondrous part of life is not knowing the future. The mind can conjure so many futures that contemplation becomes folly until it happens. What of tomorrow's Nursing Homes? What is yet to come?

Looking to the past to understand the future, we cannot deny that technology has enriched our lives. But when it comes to human relationships, there never has been a substitute for personal contact—speaking, feeling, touching—to enrich the life experience.

Nursing Home care is aimed at filling that need, one which has not changed from the very beginning. But the process of giving care has changed a lot in just the last quarter of a century.

A variety of care givers now support the Nursing Home resident to provide many types of service. This care is delivered in smaller and smaller bits, spread among many personnel. Unfortunately, each new touch is a little more expensive than before. Actually, this has been the trend for all of medicine.

how much can we give?

There seems to be no limit to the number of ways we can improve patient care. What factors then actually curb our lofty ambitions for good care?

When a patient is admitted to a Nursing Home, computerization of the planning process as occurs with the Minimum Data Set, can add a great deal of information. But it adds considerably more time and requires more qualified and expensive personnel. Moreover, by the nature of its complexity and length, it appears subject to considerable error. What will it really add to the quality of life for the patient? Have we calculated the value of this effort? Is it worth the price? Are we choosing to study our patients or give them personal care?

Releasing restraints to free disabled elders is a commendable goal. However, if the result is padding the floors and the walls, putting futons on the floors for sleeping, knee and elbow protectors on frail arms, and increasing personnel to provide one-on-one care, have we placed the cost of the service beyond reasonable means?

These questions raise still others about our modern approach to health care. How much technology can we apply to the care of the elderly? Can individuality endure when we apply the same rules and regulations to each case? Will providers be capable of adapting their ways to meet the challenges of new technology? When will the private funds of millions of retired persons be exhausted in our quest for meeting new standards? What have we to show for our efforts so far? Where's the proof that what the regulators are planning is viable? Are they obligated to prove the value of a new method before it becomes policy?

Then there are the moral questions that nag daily at our sensitivities—about dying, resuscitation, major surgery, life-sustaining methods, and euthanasia.

euthanasia

Morality is at the heart of the euthanasia issue. A debate goes on in our country but not in the Netherlands. There, euthanasia is a legitimate and common end for incurable terminal diseases. We are probably not far from it in this country since public opinion supports the concept. No doubt, the debate will be loud and grisly but a cost crisis may hurry it up.

Even now we should probably include some euthanasia clause as an option in our "**BODYRIGHTS**" documents.

As is true for all new medical methods, there is great potential for abuse here. Before it is suitable and safe for the public, there will be many cases before the Courts testing the limits of the law. The very personal nature of dying is not suited to generalizations or grocery-store delivery. Once again we may find our prejudices showing.

Along with euthanasia, there are many other questions yet to be resolved as we look to tomorrow and the paths we may have to take.

direction

The key is direction—a clear understanding of what we want to accomplish, an achievable goal, a reasonable effort that will not overburden the care-giver or pauper the patient.

Many more of the elderly will soon be upon us. In addition, poor immigrants are flooding our borders. The full devastation of the AIDS epidemic has yet to be felt. Drug-abuse-induced disability will bring multitudes to Nursing Home doors at very young ages. What have we planned for them? How will this affect the elderly?

The great health issues of the day are not really Nursing Home questions but questions of national goals for appropriate health care for all citizens.

national health

For thirty years now, the practice of medicine has slowly been transferred from the hands of physicians. The Federal Government is preparing to take over the medical care of the entire nation. A private medical sector will survive, but it will be heavily regulated. In retrospect, the process seems to have been inevitable.

change

The forces that drive us are mutating even as we adapt. Even now attitudes about death and terminal illness are changing with media exposure to these emotional issues. Will there be time to accommodate change? Will individuals and institutions soon be forced to choose sides?

The treatment of the elderly will submit to time as history has shown. Changing values and a new morality will one day result in far different solutions and options than today. For those who go on, the prospects are numerous. The frontier of aging is ever born anew.

SUMMARY:

As quickly as science has advanced to new frontiers of treatment, so has been the evolution of our ideas and attitudes about aging. Management of the advanced elderly will spark new debate that will see many new systems emerge. A new flood of Nursing Home residents is looming on the horizon—a clear challenge for tomorrow.

OPTIONS:

- Plan ahead for as many circumstances as you can envision in writing directives to your physician. Tomorrow will come.
- Planners of tomorrow will have the options of more technology or returning to simpler methods of caring.

Chapter 22

THE LAST ACT

preserving "BODYRIGHTS"

Old English prayer:
Now I lay me down to sleep
I pray the Lord my soul to keep
If I should die before I wake
I pray the Lord my soul to take.

Twentieth Century addendum:
And if I wake without my mind
God bless the choice my keepers find.

By now you realize that there is one more important thing to be done, **one last act** to perform. Protect your "**BODYRIGHTS**."

why?

Imagine that your body is alive and functioning but your mind cannot communicate with it or any other person, not for a week, a month, or for many years. Imagine modern medical science keeping your body alive but being unable to restore your mind. Imagine your family and friends and how they might feel.

What would you want to do with your body? What would you want to say to your family, your friends, your doctor? Whose pleas will your doctor heed, or whose side will the Courts take?

You can make a statement. You can protect your "BODYRIGHTS," the rights you exercise when you advise others of what you want to do when your tongue can no longer speak your mind.

While the mind is sound, it is crucial to enact a treatment plan. **Protect your body from the public keepers!**

This is true for a Nursing Home resident who is still rational. It is true for everyone else who is of legal age and does not know his future!

a will

When we have something of worth and desire to leave it to another who may outlive us, we write a **Living Trust** or a **Last Will and Testament**. Like everything else in our lives, these must be processed legally, as the Government strives to take the last measure of tax. We all know the consequences of dying rich, the attraction our assets have for so many, and the testamentary battles that can rage.

a body

Although dying bodies, or more precisely, bodies without a legally functioning mind, have not the same attraction, the rewards of caring for them can be great, especially if insurance money or a large estate is available to pay for intense medical care. There can be a tangle of claims and rights. There is much here to be determined and adjudicated, hence the long deliberations in the Courts about dying.

instruments

There are several ways of instructing others in the care of your body if and when your mind is no longer in control. **"BODYRIGHTS"** indicate we each have the right to protect our own body in these circumstances.

At the present time there are at least three legal instruments, called **Advanced Directives,** which may be recognized differently from State to State. They are written declarations, with one exception, **The Family Consent Laws**. More than one type may be useful to implement your wishes. Samples are given in **Appendix G**.

I. THE DURABLE POWER OF ATTORNEY FOR HEALTH CARE

This may be the most effective instrument for most patients. The patient appoints an agent to act in his behalf, in the event he should be declared **mentally incompetent** because of illness or injury. The agent can then make health care decisions as if the patient himself were speaking. Instructions given beforehand are meant to guide the agent in his choices of health care. If the agent is unclear, or waivering, or emotionally incapable of making hard choices in critical situations, this can be a disaster. **Choose your agent carefully and this directive will work very well.**

Every kind of medical situation can be managed by this directive. It only applies at times when the patient cannot make his own decisions. If the patient recovers his mental capacities, then once again he directs his own care.

II. DIRECTIVE TO PHYSICIANS

This can be one of several documents that specifies the kinds of treatments that the patient does not want, as well as those he may choose to elect.

The Living Will

Called by many names, **"Medical Directive," "Natural Death Declaration," or "Life Support System Affidavit," The Living Will** is a declaration regarding the use of life-sustaining procedures in the event of an incurable illness which is considered terminal. In many States there is a **"Natural Death Act"** which governs the use of this type of directive.

The critical limitation is the need to be declared "terminally ill." Many medical conditions can be treated by various methods and may not technically be "terminal" if treatment is given. This is a serious drawback to **The Living Will**.

Directives for Care

These are often used in Nursing Homes to indicate treatment wishes about a number of issues, such as CPR, tube feedings, intravenous fluids, antibiotics, pain medications, etc,. Many institutions have expanded the list to include even more options.

Not necessarily related to a terminal condition, these directives can be quite specific about treatment and expand the concept of **Physician Directives**. A simple form might relate primarily to the use of CPR for example. Expanded forms may specify the full range of treatments that may be rejected or accepted. See **Appendix G** for examples.

No doubt, more and more types of Directives will become common, amplifying the choices for patients in a number of medical conditions. Proper execution is essential and this may yet need some clarification in the Courts.

III. FAMILY CONSENT LAWS

These are newer applications of the law to include verbal instructions given to family members, not ever having been written beforehand. Some adjudications have been made on this basis and this newer concept is expanding. Clearly the weakest declarations because they are oral, they are a last resort for families with nothing else to fall back upon.

requirements

Every State has its own version of these legal instruments. You must conform to State law. **Very inexpensive forms are readily available.**

An attorney is not necessary.

Witnessing and Notarization are spelled out carefully. Be sure you comply with requirements.

No one must sign any of these documents. You can refuse.

Revocation laws are also clear. **You are permitted to change your mind!**

reform

Many lawyers feel that this whole area of the law is in need of review and reform. They expect to see other laws expanded widely in the next few years. **The Patient Self-Determination Act**, discussed in **Chapter 7**, will focus attention on these options in all treatment settings. Because it will touch patients whose illness is still unclear and whose options are too numerous to count, it may generate great confusion in the acute hospital situation. Further clarification and other directives are likely to follow.

All of these instruments are an extension of the right of American citizens to free choice.

These documents can be used to circumvent a lengthy judiciary process and costly methods of our Court system where several roles conflict regarding appropriate treatment.

Everyone needs a method to protect his **BODYRIGHTS**. Especially when today's activists, usually third parties, are entangling themselves in test cases to affect the process of medical care. They often act in behalf of the disabled or incompetent patient, professing a special insight into what should be done.

The cost of taking advantage of the available instruments is very low. No one need be rich to protect his "BODYRIGHTS."

the rest are fools

Should you be someone who as yet has failed to protect yourself or a loved one, **DO IT NOW! SET DOWN THIS BOOK AND FIND THE DOCUMENTS THAT WILL PROTECT YOU FROM THE PRESENT SYSTEM.**

Look carefully at Appendix G. Find out about the proper documents in your State (whether statutory or as recognized by the Courts of the State). Waste no time. Go to your local hospital, neighborhood bookstore, County Medical Society, your Family Doctor or your Attorney. Gain the right to decide your own fate, should you be rendered mentally incompetent.

CAUTION: There are no guarantees. Even the best-laid plans may be thwarted by the Courts, an unfaithful agent, your physician, or your family!

the agent

If you designate an agent or person to act in your behalf, find someone who is likely to survive you and who will be available. You must have complete trust in his ability to see that your wishes are carried out.

If a family member has problems in making decisions, he should never agree to serve in the capacity of agent. It is better to keep away from the medical battlefields where wounds are unpredictable and choices seem like no choice at all. Winning may seem impossible!

The Nursing Home resident about whom you are concerned will hopefully have expressed opinions and will have already signed the necessary papers upon which you may act to guarantee pre-determined wishes.

newer dilemmas

Every matter of concern to you should be addressed when writing your directives, with a view to providing protection for yourself. As mentioned already, I suspect that one day soon, **euthanasia consent** will need to be included as an option.

Needless to say, the decisions you make may not always anticipate the realities of terminal illness. The complexity of choices may carry beyond the scope of what was expected. You can only do your best to be responsible and your agent can only do his best.

timing is critical

As with all legal documents, the time specified by law during which they are effective is critical. Most documents expire in five to seven years. If you have already signed such a directive, review the expiration date. **Do it now! Keep current!**

SUMMARY:

The first order of business for a mindful person is to protect his BODYRIGHTS. Spell out in detail what you do and do not want to happen to your body when you no longer have control. Nursing Home residents should review what they have done and get current with the times.

OPTIONS:

- Establish a Durable Power of Attorney for Health Care or Directive to Physicians, including A Living Will or more. See that family members do the same. Provide copies to those who need to know.
- Spell out your wishes in detail if they are important to you.
- Be sure your latest directives are still in effect, not having expired under statutory limits. Check the dates!
- Keep a card in your wallet or purse to signify you have written such Directives.

APPENDIX A

NURSING HOME ORGANIZATIONAL CHART (EXAMPLE)

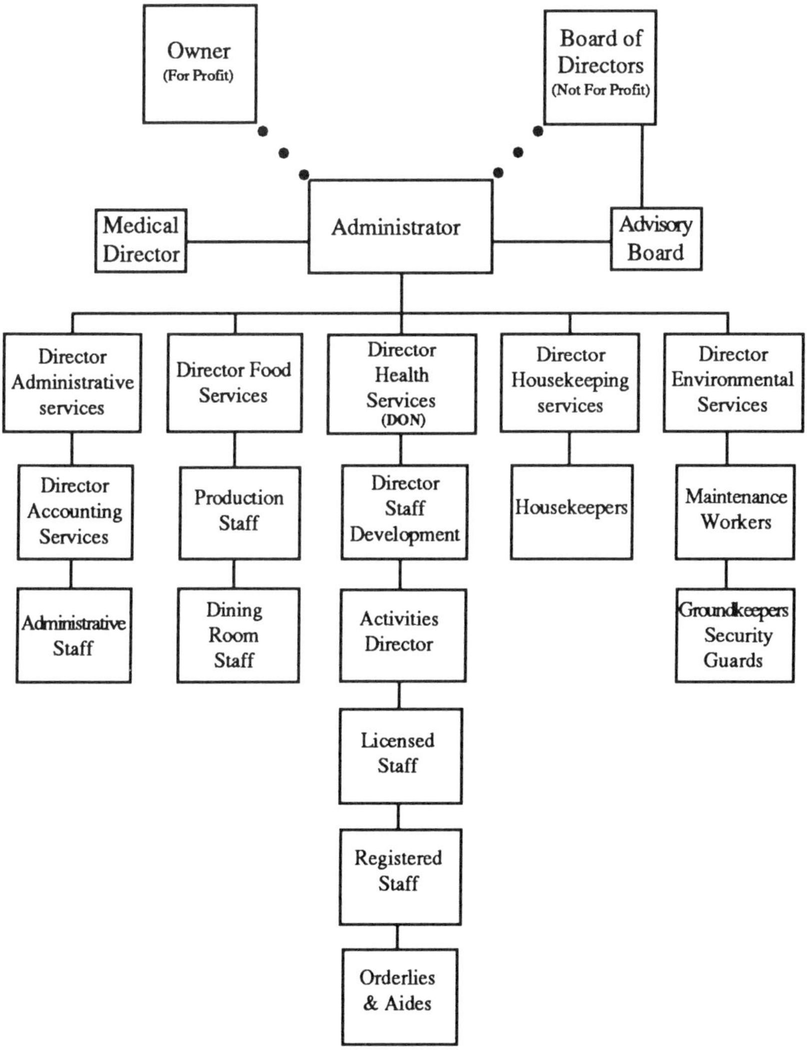

Standing Committees (most department heads and consultants)

- Utilization Review
- Quality Assurance
- Infection Control
- Pharmacy
- Fire and Safety

APPENDIX B

STAFF MEMBERS AND THEIR ROLES
typical job descriptions

Health Care Administrator

Qualifications: Graduate degree in business, public or hospital administration or in social work with proven experience in one or more of these areas. In most States must have a license as a Nursing Home Administrator.

Duties: Administers, directs, and coordinates all activities of the facility in accordance with policies established by the Owner/ Board of Directors.

Directs and coordinates all departments and services.

Supervises management of the physical plant.

Is responsible for hiring, training, supervising, and discharging supervisory staff.

Represents the facility to individuals, other organizations, and the public.

Director of Nursing Services (DON)

Qualifications: The Director of Nursing Services shall be a Registered Nurse with a current license.

Duties: Plans, organizes, directs and evaluates nursing services to meet the total needs of the patients in the health care facility.

Recruits, hires, evaluates and terminates all nursing personnel.

Prepares staff work schedules, supervises charge nurses and evaluates the performance of the nursing staff.

Oversees auxiliary personnel rendering patient-care services.

Assists in preparation of the budget.

Directs nurses' training and staff inservice education and orientation.

Attends all committee meetings.

Maintains friendly relationships with patients and residents, their families, friends and interested persons and\or groups in the community.

Medical Director

Qualifications: A licensed Medical Doctor, usually with experience in Nursing Home care, and preferably Board Certified in Geriatrics.

Duties: Responsible for planning, directing, and evaluating all medical aspects of the resident care, including review of all medical practices.

Coordinates all medical activities with the Director of Nursing Services.

Meets with policy committees, Utilization Review Committee, the Quality Assurance Committee, and other staff or administrative committees.

Consults and advises administration regarding policies, levels of care, procedures, and programs.

Often acts as attending physician and conducts a clinic for residents.

Licensed Staff (R.N., L.V.N.)

Qualifications: A State license (R.N., L.V.N.)

Duties: The Charge Nurse shall be responsible for the total nursing needs of patients and shall supervise the nursing staff assigned to her. Other Licensed Staff shall perform the duties of licensed personnel.

Insures the provision of an attractive, clean, orderly and safe patient environment.

Attends and participates in monthly staff meetings and inservice education.

Supervises the admission and discharge of patients.

Makes routine rounds on residents.

Implements physician orders and communicates changes in the patient's condition to the physician and family.

Administers medications, performs treatments, tests and other diagnostic work as ordered by the physician.

Maintains accurate health records.

Director of Nurses' Training

Qualifications: Registered Nurse

Responsibilities: Organize and implement the orientation and inservice education program for all nurse assistants and shall provide the State-required inservice education for all employees directly involved in health care.

Certified Nurse Assistant (CNA)

Duties: Provide direct patient care under the supervision of a licensed nurse.

Assists patients in the activities of daily living.

Maintains patient living area by changing and making beds, cleaning bedside equipment, doing personal laundry, etc.

Observes and reports changes in patients' physical and mental health.

Assists patients in participating in all planned activities.

Charts in the medical record.

Answers patient call lights.

Director of Administrative Services

Responsible for management and coordination of business office functions and assisting the Administrator in planning organizing, directing, evaluating and controlling.

Maintains personnel records and prepares the payroll.

Bills for Medicare and Medicaid.

Medical Records Designee

Maintains the records according to the policies and procedures established by the facility.

Compiles statistics as requested.

Oversees chart organization and completion of the records, including admission records, reports, and discharge records.

Director of Activities

Duties: Provide a balanced program of recreational activity which is adapted to the needs and abilities of the patients.

Designs and plans diversified schedules of recreation.

Utilizes volunteers.

Arranges special outings.

Prepares a monthly Calender of Events.

Maintains proper documentation of resident interests and activities.

APPENDIX C

THE USUAL NURSING HOME ADMISSIONS PACKAGE

Many documents are included in the typical admissions package. In addition each institution has its own forms and conditions peculiar to its circumstances. The following are commonly used:

- Contract for Services (Admission Agreement)
- Medicare and Medicaid Contract
  - Rates and charges
  - Transfers and discharges
  - Rules of the facility
  - Consent to treatment
  - Safekeeping
  - Photographs
  - Fee schedule
  - Theft and loss prevention
  - Medical information disclosure
- Patient Information Sheet
  - Next of Kin
  - Emergency Care Information
  - Insurance information
  - Mortuary Information
  - Tissue Organ Donor Information
- Minimum Data Set (MDS)
- Patient Bill of Rights
- Dental Agreement (resident must be examined every six months)
- Medicare A Information (if applicable)
- SNF Determination on Admission
- SNF Determination on Continued Stay
- Nursing Facility Resident Assessment (OBRA Requirement)
- Advanced Directives
  - The Durable Power of Attorney for Health Care
  - A Living Will
  - CPR Information
  - Emergency Life Support Services
  - Directive to Physicians Regarding Treatments
  - Directive to Physicians Regarding Intensity of Care
- Admission and Discharge Summary Sheet
- Notice Regarding Separate and Community Property
- AIDS Testing Consent
- Pharmacy Agreement (responsible party authorization)
- Admission and Discharge Notification Form

APPENDIX D
PATIENT RIGHTS (Simplified OBRA Version)

By law a copy of Patient Rights must be provided to patients and\or their guardian upon admission and must be prominently displayed in the facility. Of course, Civil Rights afforded by the Constitution remain in effect.

Although Nursing Homes interpret these rights somewhat differently and spell them out in detail, the following is a simplified version of basic rights.

Patients have a right:

to knowledge
- of their rights
- of their medical condition including changes
- of facility policies
- of costs
- of financial relationships with other providers
- of roommate
- of transfer

to health care
- which provides cleanliness
- which provides good food
- which provides respect
- which is free of abuse
- which permits individual habits including alcohol or tobacco
- which provides protection
- which provides confidentiality

to choice
- of physician
- of pharmacist
- of consultants
- of treatments
- of terminal care

to activities
- of managing personal affairs
- of visitation by friends and family
- of association
- of participation in social activities
- of complaining without fear

of access
- to privacy
- to mail
- to telephone
- to clothing and personal effects

to refuse
- to work
- to be restrained
- to be a research participant
- to be photographed

Patient rights may be denied or limited for good cause and only if authorized by law. Reasons for denial or limitation of such rights shall be documented by the attending physician in the patient's health record.

Nursing Homes implement these rights within their facility according to their own interpretation. Ask your Nursing Home when you have specific questions about their policies.

APPENDIX E

THE PATIENT SELF-DETERMINATION ACT OF 1990 (EFFECTIVE 1 DECEMBER 1991)

This Federal Act applies to not only Nursing Homes, but Hospitals, HMO's, Home Health Organizations, and Hospice. It requires:

At the time of admission (or initiation of the program) all adult individuals receiving care must be given written policies and procedures regarding;

—Individual rights

—The right to accept or refuse medical or surgical treatment

—The right to formulate **Advanced Directives**

Policies for implementing these rights must be given in writing.

This information must be documented in the medical record.

There must be no discrimination on the basis of the choices made.

All rights must comply with State Laws whether statutory or as recognized by the Courts.

The facility must educate the staff and community they serve about this law.

(NOTE)

Advanced Directives mean written instructions, either a Durable Power of Attorney for Health Care or a Living Will.

APPENDIX F

RESTRAINT POLICIES

Restraint policies are developed individually by each institution and may vary somewhat. Their general content is the same. They are intended to minimize harm to patients by instructing staff about their proper use.

- The physician must write an order specifying the type of restraints to be used, the indications for use, and the duration of use.

- Orders are not in effect for an indefinite period of time, but are reviewed each time before reordering.

- If restraints are ordered for more than 14 days, some Nursing Homes review the matter in committee.

- Care must be used in the proper application.

- Prolonged use should be avoided.

- The least restrictive device should be used.

- Documentation is required about the type of restraints used, when they were applied and removed, how often the patient was checked, and whether any adverse effects were noted.

- When limb restraints are used, wrists and ankles should be padded to prevent abrasions. Mittens may avoid the need for wrist restraints. Vests should be applied over hospital gowns. When patients are sitting at a table, they should be unrestrained unless there is a specific reason.

- When siderails are used to keep a patient from getting out of bed, a vest or other restraint will help to prevent crawling over the rails.

(Please refer to Chapters 9 & 21)

APPENDIX G

BODYRIGHTS DOCUMENTS
Samples of Advanced Directives

DURABLE POWER OF ATTORNEY FOR HEALTH CARE

I,____
hereby appoint ______________________________________(agent's name)
____(address)
as my agent to make health care decisions for me if and when I am unable to make my own health care decisions. This gives my agent the power to consent to giving, withholding or stopping any health care, treatment (including life-sustaining treatment), service, or diagnostic procedure. I specifically authorize my agent to make decisions for me about artificially supplied nutrition and hydration (tube feeding). My agent also has the authority to talk with health care personnel, get information, and sign forms necessary to carry out these decisions.

If the person named as my agent is not avilable or is unable to act as my agent, then I appoint the following person(s) to serve in the order listed below:

(alternate agents)
1. (NAME)
ADDRESS

2. (NAME)
ADDRESS

Sample

By this document I intend to create a power of attorney for health care which shall take effect upon my incapacity to make my own health care decisions and shall continue during that incapacity.

I have discussed my wishes with my agent, and he or she shall make all health care decisions on my behalf, including decisions to withhold or withdraw all forms of life-sustaining treatment, including artificially administered hydration and nutrition.

My particular wishes are:
(treatment options)____

by signing here I indicate that I understand the purpose of this document.

I sign my name to this form on (date) _______________

at:____(address)

________________________________(SIGNATURE)

Witness Statement, Signature, and Date
Witness Statement, Signature, and Date
or
Notary Public Acknowledgement

(Sample Only—Obtain legal form for your State)

LIVING WILL
DECLARATION

Declaration made this_____day of__________________(month, year).
I,__(DECLARER'S NAME)______________________being of sound mind, willfully and voluntarily direct that my dying shall not be artificially prolonged under the circumstances set forth in this declaration.

If at any time I should have an incurable injury, disease, or illness certified to be a terminal condition by two (2) physicians who have personally examined me, one (1) of whom shall be my attending physician, and the physicians have determined that my **death is imminent** and will occur whether or not life-sustaining procedures are utilized and where the application of such procedures would serve only to artificially prolong the dying process, I direct that such procedures be withheld or withdrawn, and that **I be permitted to die naturally** with only the administration of medication, the administration of food and water, and the performance of any medical procedure that is necessary to provide comfort, care or alleviate pain. In the absence of my ability to give directions regarding the use of such life-sustaining procedures, it is my intention that this declaration shall be honored by my family and physician(s) as the final expression of my right to control my medical care and treatment.

Other Instructions:
(treatment options)____

I am legally competent to make this declaration, and I understand its full import.

Signed____________________________________

Address____

Under penalty of perjury, we state that this declaration was signed by

(NAME OF DECLARER)____________in the presence of the undersigned who, at his/her request, in his/her presence, and in the presence of each other, have hereunto signed our names and witnessed this____________day of__________________, 19___.
Further each of us, individually, states that: The declarant is known to me, and I believe the declarant to be of sound mind. I did not sign the declarant's signature to this declaration. Based upon information and belief, I am not related to the declarant by blood or marriage, a creditor of the declarant, entitled to any portion of the estate of the declarant under any existing testamentary instrument of the declarant, entitled to any financial benefit by reason of the death of the declarant, financially or otherwise responsible for the declarant's medical care, or an employee of any such person or institution.

signature____________________________________
address_____________________________________

signature____________________________________
address_____________________________________

Notary Public Acknowledgement

(Sample Only—Obtain legal form for your State)

DIRECTIVES TO PHYSICIANS

REQUEST FOR CARE (Simplified Version)

The patient and/or the legal representative request the following treatment:

1. ☐ Maximum treatment or ☐ supportive care only
2. ☐ CPR or ☐ No CPR
3. ☐ Withdrawal of all medications

____
Responsible Party

____
Physician

____
Date

PREFERRED INTENSITY OF SUPPORTIVE CARE

The patient and/or the legal representative request **supportive care only.**

I/we understand that "supportive care" means that the principle goals of treatment will be to alleviate suffering, promote comfort and preserve dignity. The following choices of therapy represent our wishes:

THERAPY	Yes	No		Yes	No
Supportive medication			Simple blood tests		
Pain medication			Invasive tests		
Blood transfusions			Chemotherapy		
Antibiotics			Kidney dialysis		
Intravenous fluids			Minor surgery		
Nasogastric fluids			Major surgery		
Hospitalization			Organ transplant		
Oxygen			Assisted breathing		
Artificial nutrition/fluids			CPR		

Other____

The following medical conditions support the intensity of care determination made above

____
____

____
Responsible Party

____
Physician

____
Date

Index

ORDER FORM

Telephone orders: Call toll free: 1 (800) 645-8723
or (805) 687-7611
Have your Visa or MasterCard ready.
Fax orders: (805) 687-6249

Postal Orders: James N. Fisher, M.D.
c/o Collective Creations by Fisher
262 Morada Lane
Santa Barbara, CA 93105

Please send ***NURSING HOME*** **OPTIONS** @ $9.25 each

Discount for Bulk Purchase

10 or more	No Tax or Shipping Charge
25 or more	10% off cover price No Tax or Shipping Charge
100 or more	20% off cover price No Tax or Shipping Charge

Number of Copies ____________

Name: ______________________________________

Address: ____________________________________

City: ______________________ State __ Zip ________
(Please add 7.75% for books shipped to California addresses)

Shipping Book Rate: $1.75 for the first book and 75 cents for each additional book (surface shipping may take three to four weeks)
Air Mail: $3.00/book
Enclosed is $____________ (payable to James N. Fisher, M.D.)

☐ Check
☐ Credit Card
Visa☐ MasterCard☐

Card Number ☐☐☐☐ ☐☐☐☐ ☐☐☐☐ ☐☐☐☐
Name on Card_________________________ Exp date__________

INTERESTED IN MEDICAL SCIENCE FICTION?
You might enjoy reading Dr. Fisher's intriguing novel about the AIDS Virus mutation of the late 1990's. ***And Into Death's Spiral*** is an insightful book about the future of Medicine. $13.90 softcover. 313 pages. $15.00 includes tax and shipping.
Please include ____ copies with my order!

CALL *TOLL FREE* AND ORDER NOW!